# Contributors

*Author*
**Mark A. Riddle, MD**
Professor of Psychiatry and Pediatrics
Johns Hopkins University School of Medicine
Baltimore, MD

*Contributing Editors*
**Jane Meschan Foy, MD, FAAP, Chair**
Professor of Pediatrics
Wake Forest University School of Medicine
Winston-Salem, NC
Chair, AAP Task Force on Mental Health, 2004–2010
Member, AAP Mental Health Leadership Work Group, 2011–present

**Rebecca A. Baum, MD, FAAP**
Clinical Assistant Professor of Pediatrics
Nationwide Children's Hospital
The Ohio State University
Columbus, OH

**Susan dosReis, PhD**
Associate Professor
University of Maryland School of Pharmacy
Baltimore, MD

**Stanley I. Fisch, MD, FAAP**
Primary Care Practice
Harlingen Pediatrics Associates
Harlingen, TX

**Lynne C. Huffman, MD, FAAP**
Associate Professor of Pediatrics
Stanford University School of Medicine
Stanford, CA

**David B. Pruitt, MD**
Professor of Psychiatry and Pediatrics
Director, Division Child and Adolescent Psychiatry
University of Maryland
Baltimore, MD

**Gloria M. Reeves, MD**
Associate Professor
Division of Child and Adolescent Psychiatry
University of Maryland School of Medicine
Baltimore, MD

**Lawrence S. Wissow, MD, MPH, FAAP**
Professor of Health, Behavior, and Society
Johns Hopkins School of Public Health
Baltimore, MD

# What People Are Saying

"This clear and well-organized volume provides an excellent and useful compendium of advice on the use of psychotropic medications in pediatric primary care. Building on strong work by the AAP over the past 15 to 20 years to develop clinical practice guidelines for primary care management of attention-deficit/hyperactivity disorder and the work of the AAP Task Force on Mental Health, this book offers clear guidance on when to use psychotropics, which to use, and what coexisting conditions and side effects the clinician should monitor."

James M. Perrin, MD, FAAP

John C. Robinson Chair in Pediatrics

MassGeneral Hospital for Children

President (2014), American Academy of Pediatrics

"This guide to pediatric psychopharmacology provides pediatric primary care clinicians, and specialists working with them, with a practical clinical resource that concisely integrates relevant current literature and significant experience. Within a helpful framework that emphasizes safety and efficacy, this book provides clear guidance on dosing, monitoring, and potential adverse reactions. It makes access to and use of the information simple, yet incredibly valuable, for the busy clinician."

Christopher J. Kratochvil, MD

Professor of Psychiatry and Pediatrics

Anna O. Stake Professor of Child Psychiatry

Associate Vice Chancellor for Clinical Research, University of Nebraska Medical Center

Vice President for Research, Nebraska Medicine

Chief Medical Officer, UNeHealth

Poomathi Sadhishkumar, MD

# Pediatric Psychopharmacology

## FOR PRIMARY CARE

## Mark A. Riddle, MD

CONTRIBUTING EDITORS

Jane Meschan Foy, MD, FAAP, Chair
Rebecca A. Baum, MD, FAAP
Susan dosReis, PhD
Stanley I. Fisch, MD, FAAP
Lynne C. Huffman, MD, FAAP
David B. Pruitt, MD
Gloria M. Reeves, MD
Lawrence S. Wissow, MD, MPH, FAAP

American Academy of Pediatrics
141 Northwest Point Blvd
Elk Grove Village, IL 60007-1019
www.aap.org

**American Academy of Pediatrics Publishing Staff**

Mark Grimes, *Director, Department of Publishing*

Peter Lynch, *Manager, Digital Strategy and Product Development*

Theresa Wiener, *Manager, Publishing and Production Services*

Amanda Cozza, *Editorial Specialist*

Linda Diamond, *Manager, Art Direction and Production*

Mary Lou White, *Director, Department of Marketing and Sales*

Linda Smessaert, *Brand Manager, Clinical and Professional Publications*

Published by the American Academy of Pediatrics

141 Northwest Point Blvd, Elk Grove Village, IL 60007-1019

847/434-4000

Fax: 847/434-8000

www.aap.org

Library of Congress Control Number: 2012939434

ISBN: 978-1-58110-275-8

eBook: 978-1-58110-996-2

EPUB: 978-1-58110-998-6

Kindle: 978-1-58110-999-3

MA0415

The recommendations in this publication do not indicate an exclusive course of treatment or serve as a standard of medical care. Variations, taking into account individual circumstances, may be appropriate.

Statements and opinions expressed are those of the author and not necessarily those of the American Academy of Pediatrics.

Every effort has been made to ensure that the drug selection and dosages set forth in this text are in accordance with the current recommendations and practice at the time of publication. It is the responsibility of the health care professional to check the package insert of each drug for any change in indications and dosage and for added warnings and precautions.

The inclusion of product names and photos in this publication is for informational purposes only and does not imply endorsement by the American Academy of Pediatrics.

The American Academy of Pediatrics is not responsible for the content of the resources mentioned in this publication. Web site addresses are as current as possible but may change at any time.

This book has been developed by the American Academy of Pediatrics. The authors, editors, and contributors are expert authorities in the field of pediatrics. No commercial involvement of any kind has been solicited or accepted in the development of the content of this publication.

9-351/1015

1 2 3 4 5 6 7 8 9 10

# Contents

# Introduction

## What Is This Book?

This book is designed to provide primary care clinicians with a practical and coherent approach to prescription and management of psychotropic medications for children and adolescents.

The book covers 4 main concepts.

- Conceptual framework
- Guiding clinical principles
- Clinical guidance about specific diagnoses and medications
- Next steps when difficulties persist

The Contents provides a detailed outline of each part. Each chapter is designed to "stand alone" so that, depending on the reader's knowledge, skills, and experience, relevant chapters and sections may be specifically utilized. Additionally, numerous resources are included in the appendixes, with an emphasis on access to electronic content from the American Academy of Pediatrics (AAP).

## Target Audience

The primary audience for this book is pediatric primary care clinicians (pediatric PCCs) who care for children and adolescents with common psychiatric disorders and mental health or behavioral problems in their outpatient practices and who prescribe and monitor medications, including

- Primary care pediatricians
- Family physicians
- Pediatric physician assistants
- Pediatric, psychiatric, and family nurse practitioners

Secondary audiences include specialists who provide consultation to primary care clinicians in performing those roles, including

- Developmental-behavioral pediatricians
- Specialists in neurodevelopmental disabilities
- Child and adolescent psychiatrists

- Specialists in adolescent medicine
- Pediatric neurologists
- Some adult psychiatrists with training in adolescent care

Another secondary audience is allied mental health professionals, who collaborate with medication prescribers and who can provide evidence-based psychotherapies and other care for children and adolescents, including

- Psychologists
- Social workers
- Nurses
- Counselors

And, finally, another important audience is those who want to understand how clinicians strategize about medication for children and adolescents, including

- Parents, guardians, and caregivers
- Families
- Youth
- Advocates
- Policy makers

# Why Now?

The need for a conceptual framework with practical guidance for pediatric psychopharmacology is critical.

- At least 8 million US youth (10%) have an impairing psychiatric disorder.[1]
- A persistent critical shortage of mental health specialists, especially child and adolescent psychiatrists (<8,000 practicing), hinders ability to meet the needs of these youth.

Pediatric PCCs are ideally suited to meet this need because of their knowledge of child development, their long-term relationships with patients and families, and the frequency with which they encounter children and teens.

There are many—about 170,000—US pediatric PCCs.

- Approximately 60,000 primary care pediatricians (Ken Shaw, AAP, communication, October 29, 2014)
- Greater than 80,000 family physicians[2]
- Approximately 2,000 pediatric physician assistants[3]

- Approximately 14,000 pediatric nurse practitioners[4]
- Approximately 12,000 youth-dedicated family nurse practitioners[5]

The AAP[6] recommends that primary care pediatricians achieve competence in initiating care for children and adolescents with attention-deficit/hyperactivity disorder (ADHD), anxiety, depression, and substance use and abuse. This raises important considerations.

- Treatment of 3 of these conditions—attention-deficit/hyperactivity disorder, anxiety, and depression—may, under certain conditions, include medication.
- Many pediatric PCCs report having insufficient knowledge, skills, and training to prescribe safe and effective psychotropic medications to youth with these conditions.
- Continuing medical education courses in pediatric psychopharmacology targeted to pediatric PCCs are rare; maintenance of certification courses are even rarer.
- Pediatric residency training in psychiatric assessment and psychopharmacology is limited, and requirements are minimal.[7]
- Child psychiatry consultation programs are forming in many parts of the country to fill these gaps by providing real-time clinical guidance to pediatric PCCs[8]; it is critical that consultants in these programs apply a framework that recognizes realities of the primary care setting.

Because of limited time and resources for obtaining new knowledge and skills, pediatric PCCs and those who train or consult with them need an approach to pediatric psychopharmacology that is coherent, practical, and sufficiently simple to meet their needs.

## Basic Principles

A few basic principles provide the foundation for all recommendations in this book, as follows:

- Evaluation and diagnosis of ADHD, common anxiety disorders, and depression in children and adolescents can be relatively simple and straightforward when a few basic guidelines are followed.
- Whenever possible, psychotropic medications should be prescribed concomitantly with, or following inadequate response to, evidence-based psychotherapies and evidence-informed pragmatic supports.
- Medications that have US Food and Drug Administration approval for the patient's diagnosis (or a similar diagnosis) are recommended, whenever possible, because these medications have met a formal standard for

efficacy and safety and generally have more available information regarding use in youth.

■ There are only a few classes of medications (eg, stimulants, $\alpha_2$-adrenergic agonists, and selective serotonin reuptake inhibitors) that need to be mastered to effectively treat most presentations of ADHD, common anxiety disorders, and depression.

■ Providing clinical, in addition to medicolegal, informed consent and assent can strengthen and help sustain a therapeutic alliance with the patient and caregivers.

■ Prescribing as few psychotropic medications as possible simplifies the task of monitoring efficacy and safety.

■ Sequential, not simultaneous, changes in medication or dosage are recommended, whenever possible.

■ Monitoring for safety is as important as monitoring for effectiveness.

■ Use of pragmatic supports can improve efficiency and effectiveness. Resources included in this book are derived from the US Food and Drug Administration as well as national organizations such as the American Academy of Pediatrics and the American Academy of Child and Adolescent Psychiatry.

■ As an important component of the continuum of mental health care, pediatric PCCs will encounter children for whom additional specialty care is required. Consultative and collaborative relationships with mental health professionals are thus important.

## What About the Future?

■ The conceptual framework and treatment strategies in this book are designed to prepare pediatric PCCs for future developments. Fortunately, new information about the safety and efficacy of existing psychopharmacologic agents will accrue, and safer and more effective medications for children and adolescents will be developed and disseminated. Based on its recent emphasis on pediatric mental health, we can anticipate that the American Academy of Pediatrics (and other professional organizations) will provide ongoing and up-to-date educational and training opportunities for interested clinicians (see Appendix C, Training Resources for Clinicians).

■ As US health care systems continue to evolve under the Affordable Care Act,[9] emphasis on value-based medicine will continue to grow. Accountable Care Organizations and similar entities that incentivize cost reduction while maximizing quality will be responsible for providing care to specific populations within a fixed total budget. Financial benefit of safe and effective medication prescribing is a key component in the effort to secure funds for necessary evidence-based mental health treatments.

■ Treatment strategies suggested in this book emphasize use of generic medications, when appropriate, and de-emphasize use of multiple medications, which can lead to added adverse effects and cost, unless clearly needed. These strategies can have the additional benefit of reducing costs while maintaining quality.

# References

1. US Department of Health and Human Services. *Mental Health: Culture, Race, and Ethnicity—A Supplement to Mental Health: A Report of the Surgeon General.* Rockville, MD: US Department of Health and Human Services; 2001. http://www.surgeongeneral.gov/library/reports. Accessed May 21, 2015

2. US Department of Health and Human Services, Agency for Healthcare Research and Quality. The number of practicing primary care physicians in the United States: primary care workforce facts and stats no. 1. http://www.ahrq.gov/research/findings/factsheets/primary/pcwork1/index.html. Publication No. 12-P001-2-EF. Reviewed October 2014. Accessed May 21, 2015

3. Freed GL, Dunham KM, Moote MJ, Lamarand KE; American Board of Pediatrics Research Advisory Committee. Pediatric physician assistants: distribution and scope of practice. *Pediatrics.* 2010;126(5):851–855

4. National Association of Nurse Practitioners. Membership. http://www.napnap.org/membership. Accessed May 21, 2015

5. Freed GL, Dunham KM, Loveland-Cherry CJ, Martyn KK; American Board of Pediatrics Research Advisory Committee. Family nurse practitioners: roles and scope of practice in the care of pediatric patients. *Pediatrics.* 2010;126(5):861–864

6. American Academy of Child and Adolescent Psychiatry Committee on Health Care Access and Economics Task Force on Mental Health. Improving mental health services in primary care: reducing administrative and financial barriers to access and collaboration. *Pediatrics.* 2009;123(4):1248–1251

7. Caspary G, Horwitz S, Singh M, et al. Graduating pediatric residents' training and attitudes vary across mental health problems. Paper presented at: Pediatric Academic Societies Annual Meeting; 2008; Elk Grove Village, IL. http://www.aap.org/en-us/professional-resources/Research/Pages/Graduating-Pediatric-Residents-Training-and-Attitudes-Vary-Across-Mental-Health-Problems.aspx. Accessed May 21, 2015

8. Gabel S, Sarvet B. Public-academic partnerships: public-academic partnerships to address the need for child and adolescent psychiatric services. *Psychiatr Serv.* 2011;62(8):827–829

9. Mechanic D. Seizing opportunities under the affordable care act for transforming the mental and behavioral health system. *Health Affairs.* 2012;31(2)376–382

# Part 1—Conceptual Framework

# CHAPTER 1

# Conceptual Framework for Prescribing Psychotropic Medications

## Background

The American Academy of Pediatrics recommends that pediatric primary care clinicians (pediatric PCCs) achieve competence in initiating care of children and adolescents with attention-deficit/hyperactivity disorder (ADHD), anxiety, depression, and substance use and abuse. Treatment of 3 of these conditions—ADHD, anxiety, and depression—may, under certain conditions, include medication. The primary purpose of this book is to offer guidance that will assist pediatric PCCs in their decision-making about the use and monitoring of psychotropic medications.

## Rationale for the Conceptual Framework

### General Rationale

The goal of this chapter is to offer a clear, rational, and evidenced-based framework for using psychotropic medications in youth with psychiatric diagnoses. This is critical because, while many clinicians are already using these medications, there remains a wide range of comfort with, confidence in, and knowledge about how these drugs are initiated, titrated, and monitored across care settings. In addition, the large number of psychotropic medications can be overwhelming, even for experienced mental health specialists. According to an expert task force comprising representatives from major international and regional (ie, American, Asian, and European) organizations, led by the European College of Neuropsychopharmacology, 108 psychotropic medications are available for prescribing (the app NbNomenclature is available at https://play.google.com/store/apps/details?id=il.co.inmanage.nbnomenclature&hl=en and https://itunes.apple.com/us/app/nbn-neuroscience-based-nomenclature/id927272449?mt=8).

Most of these drugs are Food and Drug Administration (FDA) approved for adults in the United States.

This chapter offers a unifying approach, grounded in the most up-to-date research, for the prescribing of psychotropic medications by pediatric PCCs. The intention is not to dictate practice specifics but to offer a methodological approach that can best serve a wide range of clinicians who, after completing a thorough diagnostic assessment in which medication-responsive illness is identified, must then make decisions regarding medication treatment options for youth and families. The conceptual framework is designed to simplify and organize the medications into 3 manageable and targeted groups, in accordance with the American Academy of Pediatrics mental health competencies policy statement.[1] Following is a brief description of each of the 3 groups.

## Group 1 Medications

Group 1, the most important group of psychotropic medications for pediatric PCCs, includes medications for the common psychiatric disorders: ADHD, major depressive disorder, and anxiety disorders. The best epidemiologic data indicate that greater than 80% of psychotropic medications prescribed to youth are for ADHD, anxiety, and depressive disorders.[2]

Group 1 includes all FDA-approved medications for ADHD in youth: 2 stimulants (methylphenidate and amphetamine), 2 $\alpha_2$-adrenergic agonists (guanfacine and clonidine), and a norepinephrine reuptake inhibitor (atomoxetine). It also includes all FDA-approved medications for depression in youth: the 2 selective serotonin reuptake inhibitors (SSRIs), fluoxetine and escitalopram. There are no FDA-approved medications for youth with anxiety. This is, in large part, because of a discrepancy between FDA rules regarding anxiety disorder indications and efficacy studies that have been conducted in children and adolescents with anxiety (see Evidence Supporting Efficacy later in the chapter for details). Thus, for anxiety in youth, 3 SSRIs are included—fluoxetine, fluvoxamine, and sertraline—that all have one high-quality, positive, safety and efficacy study for common anxiety disorders and FDA approval for obsessive-compulsive disorder (OCD), an anxiety-related condition.

Nine medications are in Group 1 (Table 1.1). It is important to emphasize that these are not a formulary or restricted list of possible medications. However, as described in greater detail in Appendix D, they are the only medications with high-quality scientific evidence supporting their efficacy.

Table 1.1. Group 1 Medications[a]

| Drug (Mode of Action) | Indication[b] | US FDA Approval and Approved Age, years |
|---|---|---|
| **ADHD** | | |
| Methylphenidate (stimulant) | ADHD | Yes; ≥6 |
| Amphetamine (stimulant)[c] | ADHD | Yes; ≥6 |
| Guanfacine ($\alpha_2$-adrenergic agonist) | ADHD | Yes; ≥6 |
| Clonidine ($\alpha_2$-adrenergic agonist) | ADHD | Yes; ≥6 |
| Atomoxetine (NRI) | ADHD | Yes; ≥6 |
| **CERTAIN ANXIETY DISORDERS[d] AND OCD** | | |
| Fluoxetine (SSRI) | (Anxiety) | No |
| | OCD | Yes; ≥7 |
| | MDD | Yes; ≥8 |
| Sertraline (SSRI) | (Anxiety) | No |
| | OCD | Yes; ≥6 |
| Fluvoxamine (SSRI) | (Anxiety) OCD | No Yes; >10 |
| **MAJOR DEPRESSIVE DISORDER** | | |
| Fluoxetine (SSRI) | MDD | Yes; ≥8 |
| Escitalopram (SSRI) | MDD | Yes; ≥12 |

Abbreviations: ADHD, attention-deficit/hyperactivity disorder; FDA, Food and Drug Administration; MDD, major depressive disorder; NRI, norepinephrine reuptake inhibitor; OCD, obsessive-compulsive disorder; SSRI, selective serotonin reuptake inhibitor.

[a] Evidence of efficacy, favorable adverse effect profile, and management of disorder within primary care competencies; for a detailed discussion on pediatric mental health competencies for primary care, see Committee on Psychosocial Aspects of Child and Family Health: Task Force on Mental Health, 2009.[1]

[b] Each of these disorders also has evidence-based psychosocial interventions. See Evidence-Based Child and Adolescent Psychosocial Interventions at https://www.aap.org/en-us/Documents/resilience_anxiety _interventions.pdf.

[c] Approved down to age 3, "grandfathered in."

[d] Generalized anxiety disorder, social anxiety disorder, separation anxiety disorder.

Also, these medications are relatively safe; thus, pediatric PCCs should be comfortable prescribing them and monitoring their use.

## Group 2 Medications

The second group of medications (Group 2) includes all FDA-approved medications for youth with other disorders (ie, not ADHD, anxiety, or depression). Group 2 includes 5 antipsychotics (aripiprazole, olanzapine, quetiapine, risperidone, and paliperidone) and the mood-stabilizer lithium. These medications are approved for treatment of youth with psychosis in schizophrenia, mania in bipolar disorder, and, for aripiprazole and risper-idone, "irritability" in autism spectrum disorder. However, they are most commonly used in youth to treat behavioral problems, particularly ag-gression (see Chapter 2 and the description of T-MAY in Appendix A for details). Group 2 medications have a higher risk profile than Group 1 medi-cations and are associated with more concerning acute and chronic adverse effects. Pediatric PCCs are ideally suited to monitor adverse effects of Group 2 medications. Some pediatric PCCs, for various reasons, will be involved in prescribing them.

## Group 3 Medications

The third group of medications (Group 3) includes medications not FDA approved for youth, thus not included in Groups 1 or 2. Of Group 3 medi-cations, there are about 10 that pediatric PCCs are most likely to see in their practices. These will be discussed in terms of available efficacy data and adverse effect profile. Other Group 3 medications, which are not commonly prescribed, will not be discussed, but their adverse effect profiles can be accessed via electronic media (eg, Drugs@FDA, Epocrates, Micromedex).

# Group 1 Medications for ADHD, Anxiety, and Depression

## General Rationale

Inclusion of medications that PCCs might consider basic to the management of ADHD, anxiety, and depression—Group 1 medications—was determined by available data regarding efficacy and safety.

### Evidence Supporting Efficacy

The evidence base for treatment of ADHD, common anxiety disorders (ie, generalized, social, and separation), and depression has been demonstrated in several multisite, randomized clinical trials conducted since the mid-1990s.[3-5]

The research procedure used to demonstrate efficacy of a medication is the random assignment, masked ("blinded"), placebo-controlled treatment study

(RCT). Additional design features that improve quality of RCTs include a predetermined primary outcome variable; a sufficiently large number of participants, usually estimated via a power analysis, to accurately test the efficacy hypothesis; multiple performance sites that use comparable methodology; independent funding to minimize bias (eg, in the United States, the National Institutes of Health [NIH] or another government agency); and use of independent evaluators who do not receive any information about medication adverse effects.

There is no single criterion for determining that a medication is efficacious. In adults, 2 well-designed and conducted RCTs that demonstrate superiority of active medication over placebo are the generally accepted standard used by the FDA as a necessary prerequisite for drug approval. In children and adolescents, because fewer funding resources and studies exist, the FDA sometimes relaxes this standard and approves a medication with just one large, high-quality, multicenter RCT along with other supportive data. That approach is also used by the GRADE (Grading of Recommendations, Assessment, Development and Evaluation) Work Group to evaluate treatments for children and adolescents (www.gradeworkinggroup.org).

One of the widely recognized limitations with this approach to determining efficacy is that, for both ethical and practical reasons, RCTs are short-term, while most psychotropic medications are used to treat children and adolescents with chronic disorders that often require long-term treatment. Despite this limitation, the well-designed and conducted RCT is the best method available for demonstrating efficacy.

No medications have FDA-approved pediatric indications for an anxiety disorder (except for OCD, an anxiety-related condition), in large part, because of a discrepancy between FDA rules regarding anxiety disorder indications and efficacy studies that have been conducted in children and adolescents with anxiety. The FDA requires that studies used to support an application for an indication focus on a single anxiety disorder, such as social anxiety disorder, separation anxiety disorder, or generalized anxiety disorder. In children, symptoms and diagnoses of these disorders often co-occur and change over time. Thus, several well-designed studies sponsored by the NIH have examined use of an SSRI, such as fluoxetine,[6] fluvoxamine,[7] or sertraline,[5] to treat children with 1, 2, or 3 of the common childhood anxiety disorders (social, separation, or generalized). Most commonly, participants in these studies met criteria for 2 or 3 disorders, not just 1. Therefore, the FDA did not use data from these studies to support an indication.

For a summary of efficacy data supporting use of Group 1 medications, see Appendix D.

## Evidence Supporting Safety

There is no criterion for assessing safety of medications in children and adolescents. We selected 5 parameters for assessing safety.

1. An FDA-approved pediatric indication (a proxy for a minimal standard of research data supporting short-term safety [and efficacy] of a medication for a specified indication)

2. At least 10 years on the market (a proxy for sufficient time to discover rare adverse long-term consequences and rare complications with long-term exposure [ie, greater exposure over time increases the chance to detect rare and harmful adverse effects that would not otherwise be detected in brief clinical trials])

3. Minimal overdose harm, determined by a review of available literature

4. Lack of clinically significant boxed warnings (a formal FDA proxy for rare, major adverse effects [See Chapter 3, FDA Boxed Warnings, for discussion of clinical significance.])

5. Lack of other known or potentially harmful long-term effects, determined by a review of available literature and warnings and precautions in FDA package inserts

Table 1.2 applies these safety parameters to the 4 categories of Group 1 medications.

## Specific Rationale

Group 1 medications for use in the primary care setting belong to 4 different classes of medications.

## Stimulants

Despite numerous products available on the market, just 2 are distinct stimulant chemical entities: *methylphenidate* and *amphetamine*. Available literature has not shown advantages of different racemic mixtures (D- vs DL-). Thus, different racemic preparations are considered interchangeable, except for dose. Methylphenidate and amphetamine are available in numerous release preparations that provide a treatment effect ranging from 3 to 12 hours. Those with longer time on the market and lower cost may be preferred, but that is a general comment, not a preparation-specific recommendation.

**Table 1.2. Safety Profile of Group 1 Medication Classes in Children and Adolescents**

| Safety Criteria | Stimulant | α$_2$-Adrenergic Agonist | SSRI | NRI |
|---|---|---|---|---|
| US FDA approved age, years | ≥6 | ≥6 | ≥8 | ≥6 |
| Time on market, years[a] | >50 | >30 | >25 | ≥10 |
| Overdose harm | Low | Low | Very low | Very low |
| Boxed warning (major adverse effects)[b] | Drug abuse potential | None known[e] | Suicidality | Suicidality |
| Long-term risk to health[c,d] | Possible growth deceleration | None known | None known | None known |

Abbreviations: FDA, Food and Drug Administration; NRI, norepinephrine reuptake inhibitor; SSRI, selective serotonin reuptake inhibitor.

[a] Measure of exposure in large populations; time to observe potentially harmful events.

[b] Original FDA meta-analysis for suicidality: 2% for placebo and 4% active in forced dose titration studies.[8] More recent analysis[9] shows difference of 0.67%, down from 2%.

[c] Lack of studies to assess long-term risk to health, with the exception of stimulants.

[d] Stimulants and growth deceleration data are not convincing.

[e] Immediate release (not sustained-release) clonidine is associated with acute drops in blood pressure, syncope, and even death following unintentional or intentional ingestions of more than therapeutic quantities.

## α$_2$-Adrenergic Agonists

*Guanfacine* is FDA approved for ADHD in children and adolescents. It is relatively specific to the α$_{2A}$-receptor subtype, which mediates attention and other executive functions. *Clonidine* is FDA approved for ADHD in children and adolescents. It nonspecifically interacts with α$_{2A}$-, α$_{2B}$-, and α$_{2C}$-receptor subtypes. B and C receptors mediate sedation and hypotension and bradycardia. Thus, clonidine may have a less favorable adverse effect profile than guanfacine. No direct comparative data exist regarding this issue. Also, regular (not sustained-release) clonidine is associated with acute drops in blood pressure, syncope, and even death following unintentional or intentional ingestions of more than therapeutic quantities.

## Norepinephrine Reuptake Inhibitor

Atomoxetine, a norepinephrine reuptake inhibitor, has an FDA indication for ADHD. It has more concerning FDA warnings and precautions than other medications for ADHD included in Group 1.

### Selective Serotonin Reuptake Inhibitors

Six SSRIs are marketed in the United States: fluoxetine, sertraline, escitalopram, paroxetine, citalopram, and fluvoxamine. Comments regarding the
4 SSRIs included in Group 1 are

- *Fluoxetine:* FDA indications in children and adolescents for depression
  and OCD; high-quality, NIH-sponsored study demonstrating efficacy
  for the 3 common anxiety disorders in youth[6]; first SSRI marketed in the
  United States; longest half-life, so abrupt discontinuation results in slow,
  safe fall in plasma and brain levels
- *Sertraline:* FDA indication in children and adolescents for OCD; second
  SSRI on the market; shorter half-life; best data for the 3 common anxiety
  disorders in youth,[5] thus offering alternative to fluoxetine when shorter
  half-life may be indicated (eg, for a child taking multiple medications
  with further changes likely) or when fluoxetine cannot be used because
  of interactions with metabolic isoenzymes (eg, inhibition of CYP2D6)
- *Escitalopram:* FDA indication in children and adolescents for depression;
  no clinically relevant interactions with hepatic CYP450 isoenzymes
- *Fluvoxamine:* FDA indication for OCD in youth and a high-quality,
  NIH-sponsored study demonstrating efficacy for the 3 common anxiety
  disorders in youth[7]

# Group 2 Medications

## General Rationale

In addition to prescribing and monitoring Group 1 medications, pediatric
PCCs are ideally suited to collaborate with psychiatrists and other mental
health specialists in care of children and adolescents with more severe or
uncommon disorders. They may be asked to take on partial responsibility for
monitoring therapeutic and adverse effects of a variety of other medications,
which are included in Groups 2 and 3.

Group 2 medications can be monitored in primary care settings, but, because
they generally have a more serious adverse effect profile, more complicated
monitoring requirements than Group 1 medications, or both, they tend to be
prescribed by specialists.

- Child psychiatrists
- Developmental-behavioral pediatricians
- Specialists in neurodevelopmental disabilities or adolescent medicine

- Pediatric neurologists
- Adult psychiatrists with additional training in adolescent psychiatry

Depending on an individual pediatric PCC's skills and experience and (lack of) availability of specialists for referral (especially in rural and underserved areas), some pediatric PCCs with additional training in pediatric psychopharmacology may choose to prescribe Group 2 medications.

Group 2 includes all FDA-approved medications for youth with other disorders (ie, not ADHD, anxiety, or depression). Group 2 includes 5 second-generation antipsychotics (SGAs) (aripiprazole, olanzapine, quetiapine, risperidone, and paliperidone [the active metabolite of risperidone]) and lithium, a mood stabilizer. All 5 SGAs are approved for treatment of youth with psychosis in schizophrenia; all except paliperidone are approved for mania in bipolar disorder; and only risperidone and aripiprazole are approved for "irritability" in autism spectrum disorder. However, these medications are most commonly used off-label (ie, outside FDA indications) in youth to treat behavioral problems, especially aggression. Lithium is FDA approved in youth to treat acute mania in bipolar disorder. Lithium is also used off-label to treat non-bipolar mood instability.

## Specific Rationale

### Antipsychotics

Antipsychotics can reduce severity of various major psychiatric symptoms and have a variety of effects, including

- Antipsychotic effects for hallucinations, delusions, and disorganized thinking
- Mood-stabilizing effects for mania, irritability, and mood instability
- Possible "organizing" or "calming" effects for agitation and aggressive behavior

However, of all psychotropic medications used in children and adolescents, antipsychotics have the most concerning adverse effects, including

- Daytime sedation
- Weight gain
- Elevated glucose and insulin resistance
- Elevated triglyceride and cholesterol levels
- Abnormal movements (neurologic)
- Endocrine (eg, gynecomastia, galactorrhea)

Many major adverse effects of antipsychotics—particularly weight gain, metabolic abnormalities, and involuntary movements—can develop into major health problems (eg, cardiovascular disease and its consequences, tardive dyskinesia) during long-term treatment and may not be reversible. Most disorders that may be treated with antipsychotics are chronic and generally require long-term treatment. Thus, determining risk versus benefit when initiating antipsychotics is difficult.

### Mood Stabilizers

Mood stabilizers (excluding antipsychotics) have mood-stabilizing effects and are used to treat mania, depression, irritability, and problematic mood swings in bipolar disorder and other mood disorders. Two groups of mood stabilizers are available: traditional (lithium, valproic acid [divalproex sodium], and carbamazepine) and newer anticonvulsants (eg, lamotrigine). Use of mood stabilizers (excluding antipsychotics) in youth appears to be decreasing. This may be due to one or more factors: available efficacy data is generally negative; regular monitoring of plasma levels is usually required; or the adverse effects burden is substantial.

Lithium is the only mood stabilizer included in Group 2. Lithium has an FDA indication for mania in bipolar disorder down to age 12. Available data for lithium suggest efficacy for acute mania in bipolar disorder.

Chapter 6 is devoted to a more extensive presentation of Group 2 medications, including information about individual medications.

# Group 3 Medications

### General Rationale

Group 3 includes medications not FDA approved for youth, thus not included in Groups 1 or 2. Ten Group 3 medications that pediatric PCCs are most likely to see in their practices are discussed in Chapter 7 in terms of available efficacy data and adverse effect profile. Other Group 3 medications, which are not commonly prescribed, will not be discussed, but their adverse effect profiles can be accessed via electronic media (eg, Drugs@FDA, Epocrates, Micromedex).

## Specific Rationale for 10 Medications

The author and editorial advisory group selected 10 medications in Group 3 that are commonly seen in pediatric primary care. This selection was based on expert opinion because no data are available regarding prescribing of these medications in youth. These medications, which include 4 antidepressants, an antipsychotic, a mood stabilizer, 2 anxiolytics, and 2 sleep aids, are presented in Chapter 7.

# References

1. American Academy of Pediatrics Committee on Psychosocial Aspects of Child and Family Health and Task Force on Mental Health. The future of pediatrics: mental health competencies for pediatric primary care. *Pediatrics.* 2009;124(1):410–421
2. Olfson M, Blanco C, Wang S, Laje G, Correll CU. National trends in the mental health care of children, adolescents, and adults by office-based physicians. *JAMA Psychiatry.* 2014;71(1):81–90
3. The MTA Cooperative Group. Multimodal Treatment Study of Children with ADHD. A 14-month randomized clinical trial of treatment strategies for attention-deficit/hyperactivity disorder. *Arch Gen Psychiatry.* 1999;56(12):1073–1086
4. March J, Silva S, Petrycki S, et al; Treatment for Adolescents With Depression Study (TADS) Team. Fluoxetine, cognitive-behavioral therapy, and their combination for adolescents with depression: Treatment for Adolescents With Depression Study (TADS) randomized controlled trial. *JAMA.* 2004;292(7):807–820
5. Walkup JT, Albano AM, Piacentini J, et al. Cognitive behavioral therapy, sertraline, or a combination in childhood anxiety. *N Engl J Med.* 2008;359(26):2753–2766
6. Birmaher B, Axelson DA, Monk K, et al. Fluoxetine for the treatment of childhood anxiety disorders. *J Am Acad Child Adolesc Psychiatry.* 2003;42(4):415–423
7. The Research Unit on Pediatric Psychopharmacology Anxiety Study Group. Fluvoxamine for the treatment of anxiety disorders in children and adolescents. *N Engl J Med.* 2001;344(17):1279–1285
8. Hammad TA, Laughren T, Racoosin J. Suicidality in pediatric patients treated with antidepressant drugs. *Arch Gen Psychiatry.* 2006;63(3):332–339
9. Bridge JA, Iyengar S, Salary CB, et al. Clinical response and risk for reported suicidal ideation and suicide attempts in pediatric antidepressant treatment: a meta-analysis of randomized controlled trials. *JAMA.* 2007;297(15):1683–1696

# Part 2—Practical Guidance

CHAPTER 2

# Assessment

# Overview

· · · · · ·

Pediatric primary care clinicians (PCCs), because of extensive training and vast experience in assessing medical problems, have a great deal of proficiency for assessing children's and adolescents' chronic health problems and disorders. This chapter focuses on additional knowledge and skills that are needed to conduct a mental health evaluation, including

- Recognizing symptoms
- Using rating scales
- Diagnosing common disorders
- Considering comorbid diagnoses
- Preparing a brief formulation
- Providing simple and coherent feedback to the child and family

Such an evaluation may be completed in a single session, but more commonly it will take place over time as data are gathered from the child, caregiver(s), and collateral sources and as the child's response to the pediatric PCC's initial interventions are assessed.

This chapter is divided into 3 sections.

- The first section provides general clinical guidance regarding assessment and emphasizes several basic principles, as follows. Although the presence of symptoms is important, the presence of impairment or distress is the main indicator of need for treatment, and the effect of symptoms on all aspects of the child's life should be considered, including academic development, family life, interactions with peers, participation in activities, and emotional well-being. Initial primary care intervention for problems that do not meet the threshold for diagnosis can be helpful, even as the diagnostic evaluation continues. Prior to the use of medication, evidence-based psychotherapy and, when indicated, pragmatic supports are recommended; in some cases, concurrent use of psychotherapy and medication may be considered (Chapter 3).

■ The second section provides detailed information about a variety of psychiatric disorders, including *Diagnostic and Statistical Manual of Mental Disorders, Fifth Edition* (*DSM-5*) diagnostic criteria. This level of detail can be overwhelming. The intent is not to expect the reader to memorize this material. Because pediatric PCCs care for children with a broad spectrum of symptom severity yet most of these children have 1 or 2 common disorders and mild-to-moderate symptoms, this section is meant to serve as a resource about specific diagnoses when needed for specific patients or situations.

■ The third section describes a stepwise approach to formulation and feedback. This approach emphasizes partnering with the patient and family in the decision-making process.

# General Clinical Guidance

## Prepare the Office

Pediatric PCCs face a challenging yet rewarding task. They are called on to engage in preventive, assessment, treatment, and monitoring services for children and adolescents who may present with a wide spectrum of mental health concerns. Ideally, these activities are accomplished through close collaboration between the patient, family, pediatric PCC, and office staff and will be best accomplished with advanced planning. Because of the spectrum of mental health concerns presenting to primary care, pediatric PCCs and their office staff must be able to identify and address mental health emergencies, though these scenarios will likely be uncommon. Developing standard office procedures for the management of common mental health concerns, such as anxiety, low mood, inattention, and other behavioral problems, is helpful in addressing most mental health concerns that present in the primary care setting. These procedures will likely include establishing referral guidelines for mental health services in the community as well as identification of informational materials for patients and families. Use of screening tools to identify populations at risk for mental health disorders can also be useful, especially given the ongoing stigma associated with mental health conditions, which often leads to under-identification. Prior to the implementation of screening, however, practices must identify how positive findings will be addressed. Additional information on "preparing the practice" to successfully care for children with mental health concerns can be found.[1] The American Academy of Pediatrics (AAP) practice readiness inventory (see Appendix A) also serves as an assessment tool for practices to identify strengths and gaps in the care they provide to children with mental health concerns.

## Triage for Psychiatric and Social Emergencies

Triage for psychiatric and social emergencies is an essential part of the evaluation for any mental health concern. Psychiatric and social emergencies that require immediate attention, and usually a referral for emergency evaluation and treatment, are listed in Box 2.1.

Significant parent or child concern may also constitute an emergency. For example, a child or adolescent presenting with severe panic symptoms or a first panic attack requires urgent attention. Symptoms of a panic attack, such as palpitations, feelings of choking, chest pain or discomfort, fear of losing control, or fear of dying, can be frightening to a child and caregiver(s). Pediatric PCCs and their office staff must therefore consider both the type and severity of symptoms, as well as the level of distress and impairment, when defining emergency and urgent situations.

If the initial evaluation reveals that the presenting problem is not an emergency, proceeding with an evaluation that follows the sequence described below is recommended.

**Box 2.1. Psychiatric and Social Emergencies in Pediatric Primary Care**

| Psychiatric Emergencies |
| --- |
| • Suicidality |
| • Serious threat of violence by the child or adolescent |
| • Psychosis |
| • Acute alcohol or substance intoxication or withdrawal |

| Social Emergencies |
| --- |
| • Sexual or physical abuse |
| • Threat of violence to the child |
| • Family or social circumstances that threaten safety of the child/adolescent (eg, domestic violence) |
| • Inadequate family resources that pose urgent health or safety risks |

## Assess Symptom Severity

In addition to determining level of functional impairment, all clinicians struggle with determining the clinical threshold of symptom severity when deciding on a diagnosis and determining whether to initiate a specific treatment. A familiar example in pediatric primary care is attention-deficit/hyperactivity disorder (ADHD). All 18 symptoms of ADHD in the *DSM-5* include the term *often,* but there is no specific definition of *often.* Comparable examples of the struggle with threshold in general medicine include diagnosis and treatment of pain and insomnia.

Parent reports and self-reports can provide useful information about a child's symptoms and their severity, are useful in determining diagnostic threshold, and are useful during "watchful waiting." Among the many available reporting tools, the following generally incorporate current *DSM* criteria and are available as open-access tools:

- *ADHD:* NICHQ Vanderbilt Assessment Scale for parents and teachers at www.nichq.org/childrens-health/adhd/resources/vanderbilt-assessment-scales (see Appendix A)
- *Anxiety:* Screen for Anxiety Related Disorders (SCARED), parent and child versions, at www.psychiatry.pitt.edu/research/tools-research/assessment-instruments (see Appendix A)
- *Depression:* Patient Health Questionnaire-9 (PHQ-9) Modified for Teens (see Appendix A)

Beyond documentation of the total score on an assessment tool, the pediatric PCC can ask about the level of impairment and distress associated with symptoms to decide whether medication is warranted.

## Emphasize Function

Assessment of functioning is imperative, both to determine if the severity of child's symptoms meet diagnostic criteria and to formulate goals for treatment. Primary care–friendly tools in the AAP mental health toolkit include the performance section on the Vanderbilt Assessment Scale for ADHD and the Strengths and Difficulties Questionnaire (SDQ) (see Appendix A). In general, a child who has a mental health disorder and has severely impaired functioning will need care in the mental health specialty system. For children who are less impaired, the pediatric PCC and family can decide whether to engage a specialist or the mental health system (or both). Medication usually is not recommended for symptomatic treatment of children without *clinically significant functional impairment.*

## Assess Sleep Pattern

Inadequate sleep can cause distractibility, restlessness, worry, irritability, and low mood—all symptoms which may masquerade as symptoms of mental health conditions. Sleep problems can be secondary to various environmental stressors (particularly family turmoil), excessive responsibilities and activities (eg, job, athletics, homework), procrastination, or socializing (actually or virtually).

*Disrupted sleep* can be a symptom of a mental disorder or can exacerbate a mental disorder.

Inquiry regarding sleep includes determining the child's quantity and quality of sleep, satisfaction with sleep, sleep hygiene, and sleep schedule. An important element of the history is asking a youth whether she can sleep when she wants to. *Inability* to sleep—as opposed to *resistance* to sleep or poor sleep hygiene—may be more likely to suggest a psychiatric origin or a sleep disorder. Table 2.1 summarizes sleep requirements at various ages during childhood and adolescence.

If there are sleep concerns, a sleep log completed over a 2-week period can be helpful in determining patterns or areas for improvement. A convenient, single-page pediatric sleep log is available at www.brightfutures.org /mentalhealth/pdf/families/ec/diary.pdf. This information, combined with other elements of the psychosocial assessment, can assist the clinician in determining whether to prioritize the sleep problem as a primary or secondary concern.

## Identify Environmental Stressors

A growing body of literature suggests that environmental factors can have short- and long-term effects on childhood mental health and can contribute

**Table 2.1. How Much Sleep Do You Need?**

| Newborns | 16–18 hours |
|---|---|
| Preschool-aged Children | 11–12 hours |
| School-aged Children | At least 10 hours |
| Teens | 9–10 hours |
| Adults | 7–8 hours |

From Centers for Disease Control and Prevention, National Center for Chronic Disease and Prevention and Health Promotion, Division of Adult and Community Health. CDC features: are you getting enough sleep? http://www.cdc.gov/Features/Sleep. Updated April 14, 2014. Accessed May 13, 2015.

to a decline in both physical and mental health into adulthood. These adverse childhood experiences (ACEs) include exposure to poverty, abuse, family disruption, domestic violence, parental mental health disorders, and substance abuse. Mental and physical effects of ACEs appear to be cumulative, especially in the absence of protective factors and with prolonged exposure, with higher numbers of ACEs associated with more significant impairment. More information on ACEs and the ACE Score Calculator can be found at www.acestudy.org/ace_score.

In addition to the potential for long-terms effects, ACEs and other significant stressors can cause more immediate symptoms that may mimic those of ADHD, anxiety, and depression. These stressors may include single incidents (eg, car crash), ongoing trauma (eg, exposure to domestic violence), or a combination of single and ongoing stresses (none of which might alone be considered "trauma").[2]

Simple surveillance questions that can be incorporated into a standard visit include, "Since the last time I saw you, has anything really scary or upsetting happened to you or your family?" and "Are there ever times that you worry you won't have enough food to eat or a safe place to stay?" For children younger than 8 years, the analogous questions should be asked to parents (ie, "Since the last time I saw your child, has anything really scary or upsetting happened to your child or anyone in your family?"). The Safe Environment for Every Kid (SEEK) questionnaire, available at www.ncbi.nlm.nih.gov /books/NBK117231/bin/appc-fm1.pdf can be used to screen for many types of environmental stressors.

The pediatric PCC's clinical judgment, combined with the history provided by the patient and family, is essential in determining whether a response qualifies as a clinically relevant stressor. An indication that the child's safety is compromised indicates an urgent need for intervention.

## Screen for Substance Abuse

Substance use and experimentation are very common among youth. According to the Centers for Disease Control and Prevention, approximately 25% of high school–aged youth report they have bought, sold, or been given drugs on school grounds in the past 6 months (www.cdc.gov/features /YRBS). Thus, for preteens and adolescents, screening for substance abuse is recommended. The CRAFFT (car, relax, alone, forget, friends, trouble) substance abuse screening questionnaire is a validated, brief pediatric screening tool recommended for use in the primary care setting (www.ceasar-boston .org/clinicians/crafft.php).

Substance abuse and posttraumatic stress disorder (PTSD) may co-occur with other mood or behavioral disorders (eg, anxiety, depression, ADHD). Complex psychopathology may require further mental health consultation for diagnostic evaluation or incorporation of specific psychosocial treatments (or both). It is important to note that there are no US Food and Drug Administration–approved pediatric medications for either substance abuse or PTSD, but there are evidence-based psychosocial interventions (eg, motivational interviewing and trauma-informed cognitive behavioral therapy [CBT]).

## Differentiate New vs Exacerbation of Old or Chronic Problems

The breadth and depth of an initial evaluation of a mental health problem depends on the type of problem or presentation. Any new problem generally requires a thorough evaluation and diagnostic assessment, with consideration of symptom severity, functional impairment, family support, and available resources. An exacerbation of a previously diagnosed and generally stable problem will rarely require the same breadth and depth of assessment as a newly presenting problem.

Recurrences or exacerbations are often associated with some change in the child's environment or a transition to a new developmental stage. Identifying these issues is a good start to a problem-focused approach to treatment. Understanding how the present episode differs from past episodes can provide a clue as to how much new assessment is required or whether a different treatment is needed.

## Inquire About Prior Evaluations and Prior and Current Treatments

Obtaining information about previous evaluations and interventions can be useful in understanding what has, and more importantly, what has not been helpful for the child in the past. The child's and family's understanding of prior evaluations and diagnoses, as well as prior and current medications, may also influence their response to the evaluation process. Prior positive experience usually makes the current clinician's work easier; prior negative experience may lead to resistance, which can be better managed when the pediatric PCC is aware of this aspect of the child's history. Inquiry about prior and current treatments should include over-the-counter and complementary and integrative medication approaches, in part because some of these medications (eg, nutritional supplements that include the stimulant β-methylphenylethylamine or St. John's wort) may interact with prescription medications.

## Overview of Assessment of Common Disorders

Complexity of assessment of a mental health disorder depends on several factors, including (1) the proportion of salient symptoms that can be observed by caregivers and other informants, (2) the number of other relevant disorders on the differential diagnosis list, (3) the effect of environmental stressors, particularly in families affected by social determinants of health, and (4) contributing and confounding problems, such as substance abuse and medical illness. Attention-deficit/hyperactivity disorder can be straight-forward to diagnose because the symptoms of ADHD are generally observable by multiple informants (eg, parents, teachers) in multiple settings (eg, school, home). Nonetheless, ADHD can be confused with intellectual, language, and learning difficulties and may also be confused with anxiety or the effects of adverse life experiences (or both). Also, differentiating normal activity, impulsivity, and inattention from ADHD can be very difficult in preschool-aged children.

For the evaluation of internalizing disorders (eg, anxiety and depression), separate interviews of the child and caregiver(s) are recommended. This is because the child may not want to disclose to or worry a caregiver and vice versa. In addition, the caregiver may not be aware of the child's worries or negative cognitions. Separate child and caregiver rating forms are recommended.

Although anxiety and depression are both considered internalizing conditions, many symptoms of anxiety can be observed or easily elicited. Physical symptoms (eg, abdominal pain, muscle tension) are common in children with anxiety[6] and are familiar to pediatric PCCs. Other symptoms—such as avoiding social situations or phobic stimuli or entering the parents' bedroom or bed at night in response to separation concerns—are either reported by the child to the parent(s) or are readily observed by parents. When eliciting the patient's worries and internal distress, asking open-ended questions is preferred. For example, "What do you worry about?" may yield more information and is more likely to start a dialogue than asking, "Do you worry?" A response to an initial open-ended question can be followed with, "Tell me more about that." or "How is that a problem for you?"

The list of differential diagnoses for a specific anxiety disorder (eg, generalized anxiety disorder) includes all other specific anxiety disorders (eg, panic disorder, social anxiety disorder [SoAD], separation anxiety disorder [SAD], simple phobia), as well as PTSD, bereavement, depression, and oppositional defiant disorder. In addition, personality traits, such as introversion or neuroticism, may be salient.

Depression may be difficult to diagnose because demoralization, grief, and "adjustment disorder," which are common in children and adolescents, can mimic symptoms of depression. Parsing depression from these other conditions requires time and patience.

When differential diagnosis is complex, the pediatric PCC and family may choose to involve a mental health specialist in the assessment process. In most communities, licensed nonmedical mental health specialists (eg, clinical social workers, psychologists) are more accessible than psychiatrists. Some nonmedical mental health specialists are qualified to assist in assessment and diagnosis of children and adolescents with mental health problems and may be integrated into the primary care clinical team. In addition to confirming a diagnosis, this nonmedical specialist can provide psychosocial treatment and facilitate the pediatric PCC's consultation with a child and adolescent psychiatrist, as needed, to assist with medication decisions.

## Determine if Medication Is an Appropriate Treatment

It is important to recognize medication-responsive disorders (ie, disorders for which, at a minimum, there is sufficient evidence of a clinically meaningful reduction of symptom severity in response to medication) to assure that children who may benefit from medication are offered a trial and to prevent needless use of medication in children who will not benefit from such treatment.

Still, even with an accurate diagnosis and evidence-based treatments, there is no completely sensitive and specific way to determine which individual child will respond to medication or any other evidence-based therapy for psychiatric disorders; nor is there a way to predict who will experience treatment adverse effects or what type of adverse effect may emerge.

Uncertainty underlying these issues presents clinical challenges for the prescribing pediatric PCC. A relatively simple approach to assessing whether to recommend medication is outlined in Box 2.2. It emphasizes

- Symptom severity and duration
- Impairment and distress
- Differentiation from "normal"
- Prior or concurrent evidence-based behavioral therapies

This approach approximates the American Psychiatric Association *DSM-5* in essential components or criteria and practice guidelines for behavioral therapies.

**Box 2.2. Assessing Whether to Prescribe Medication**

1. Does the child have *sufficient* symptoms to support a syndrome or disorder?
2. Have the symptoms been present for a *sufficient* period?
3. Is the child experiencing *sufficient* impairment, distress, or both from the symptoms in ways that negatively affect academic development, family life, interactions with peers, participation in activities, or emotional well-being?
4. Is this disorder *sufficiently* different from normal levels of activity and impulsivity (in contrast with ADHD), worry and concern (in contrast with an anxiety disorder), or demoralization or grief (in contrast with an episode of depression)?
5. Have evidence-based therapies (eg, behavioral management training with parents for ADHD; cognitive-behavioral therapy for anxiety or depression) been *sufficient* in quality and duration, if available?

Abbreviation: ADHD, attention-deficit/hyperactivity disorder.

The term *sufficient* (or *sufficiently*) appears in each of the criteria or components in Box 2.2. Thus, the pediatric PCC must judge whether symptoms cross a threshold of severity that warrants a recommendation for medication.

In addition, age is an important consideration when deciding whether to recommend medication. In general, the younger the patient, the more important it is to consider and prescribe behavioral therapies and other psychosocial interventions before medication. This is particularly relevant for any child aged 5 and younger.

## Provide Initial Primary Care Intervention for Problems That Are Not Disorders

Many children have mild symptoms or impaired functioning without having a diagnosable disorder. Through the use of specific communication and influence skills, clinicians can be effective in decreasing the child's and family's distress and improving the child's functioning, even in the absence of a diagnosed disorder.[3] These skills can be particularly useful in primary care, either as primary treatment for mild symptoms or to help bridge treatment until referral to a specialty mental health professional can be completed. For more information, see HELP mnemonic in Appendix A.

## Recognize Need for Referral

There are also situations in which referral will be beneficial, including undiagnosed learning disabilities and complex psychosocial situations.

Youth with undiagnosed learning disabilities or cognitive impairment may also present with significant mood or behavioral problems. These problems may be related to school maladjustment (eg, symptoms occur primarily in a school setting, not at home). Parents may benefit from referral to family advocacy programs or support programs available in the school system that can provide information on obtaining learning disabilities evaluations and advocating for disability services. It can be very difficult to obtain formal assessments, as waiting times may be long, schools may be reluctant to certify the need for testing, and consultations in the community may be prohibitively expensive for some families. In the meantime, pediatric PCCs may be able to help by providing advice across a range of academic abilities, including trying to delineate the child's academic strengths and weaknesses, destigmatizing academic difficulties, troubleshooting homework habits, and identifying opportunities for additional academic support (family, peer, or school-based coaching or tutoring).

Children living with complex psychosocial situations (eg, those whose parents have mental health or substance abuse issues, cognitive impairment, or significantly impaired parenting skills or those who have been maltreated or exposed to significant childhood adversities) may also need a more thorough evaluation by a mental health professional or resources and support from the mental health system (or both). If a parent's mental illness is affecting the child's mental health, referral of the parent for his or her own care is warranted. Pediatric PCCs may want to think about how to approach these situations, including

- Finding time to talk with the parent alone
- Making sure that the parent knows the motivation of the inquiry includes help for the parent and is not just a way to help the child
- Being able to offer some practical first-line advice as well as concrete suggestions about how to approach finding care

# Assessment

## Assessment of the 3 Common Disorders

### *ADHD*

Children with possible ADHD can present to pediatric PCCs in outpatient settings, often at the urging of school personnel. Pediatric PCCs are generally skilled and experienced with the evaluation and diagnosis of a child with possible ADHD.

In the AAP clinical practice guideline "ADHD: Clinical Practice Guideline for the Diagnosis, Evaluation, and Treatment of Attention-Deficit/Hyperactivity Disorder in Children and Adolescents," the first key action statement is "The primary care clinician should initiate an evaluation for ADHD for any child 4 through 18 who presents with academic or behavioral problems or symptoms of inattention, hyperactivity, or impulsivity."[4] This includes collecting information directly from school and child care personnel who have observed the child, as well as family members (including a noncustodial parent) and youth, using a validated tool such as the NICHQ Vanderbilt Assessment Scale.

The AAP ADHD toolkit includes a wealth of useful information to facilitate the evaluation process for the child with suspected ADHD (see Appendix B). The American Academy of Family Physicians provides information and continuing medical education regarding ADHD evaluation and diagnosis through its official journal, *American Family Physician* (see www.aafp.org /afp/topicModules/viewTopicModule.htm?topicModuleId=68).

Because most pediatric PCCs are familiar with ADHD and have access to an abundance of high quality information about evaluation, this section will focus on a just a few selected topics regarding ADHD.

The most important data for diagnosing ADHD in a child reflect caregivers' and teachers' observations that are recorded and organized by structured rating scales. This is because while some children with ADHD will exhibit hyperactivity, impulsivity, or distractibility (or a combination of the 3) in the examination room, many will not. Obtaining symptom information from informants over at least a week and during various times of day strengthens the validity of the diagnosis, as symptom severity waxes and wanes over short periods.

## *DSM-5* Symptoms of Inattention in ADHD

*DSM-5 symptoms of inattention in ADHD* are listed in Box 2.3. Of note, all 9 symptoms start with the word *often*. Obviously, the meaning of often will vary among informants. Thus, it is the clinician's task to work with caregivers and teachers to clarify if a symptom is different from normal developmental expectations.

**Box 2.3. *DSM-5* Symptoms of Inattention in ADHD[a]**

a. Often fails to give close attention to details or makes careless mistakes
b. Often has difficulty sustaining attention in tasks or play activities
c. Often does not seem to listen when spoken to directly
d. Often does not follow through on instructions and fails to finish tasks
e. Often has difficulty organizing tasks and activities
f. Often avoids, dislikes, or is reluctant to engage in tasks that require sustained mental effort
g. Often loses things necessary for tasks or activities
h. Often easily distracted by extraneous stimuli
i. Often forgetful in daily activities

Abbreviation: *DSM-5, Diagnostic and Statistical Manual of Mental Disorders, Fifth Edition.*

[a] For the full *DSM-5* diagnostic criteria, see Appendix F.

Reproduced, with permission, from American Psychiatric Association. *Diagnostic and Statistical Manual of Mental Disorders.* 5th ed. Arlington, VA: American Psychiatric Association; 2013.


## *DSM-5* Symptoms of Hyperactivity and Impulsivity in ADHD

*DSM-5 symptoms of hyperactivity and impulsivity in ADHD* are listed in Box 2.4. Again, it is noteworthy that all 9 symptoms start with the word *often.* Differentiating normal developmental levels of activity and impulsivity can be challenging, particularly in young children (ie, 3- to 5-year-olds).


**Box 2.4. Simplified *DSM-5* Symptoms of Hyperactivity and Impulsivity in ADHD[a]**

| Hyperactivity |
|---|
| a. Often fidgets with or taps hands or feet or squirms in seat |
| b. Often leaves seat in situations when remaining in seat is expected |
| c. Often runs about or climbs in situations where it is inappropriate |
| d. Often unable to play or engage in leisure activities quietly |
| e. Often "on the go," acting as if "driven by a motor" |
| f. Often talks excessively |

| Impulsivity |
|---|
| g. Often blurts out an answer before a question has been completed |
| h. Often has difficulty waiting his or her turn |
| i. Often interrupts or intrudes on others |

Abbreviation: *DSM-5, Diagnostic and Statistical Manual of Mental Disorders, Fifth Edition.*

[a] For the full *DSM-5* diagnostic criteria, see Appendix F.

Reproduced, with permission, from American Psychiatric Association. *Diagnostic and Statistical Manual of Mental Disorders.* 5th ed. Arlington, VA: American Psychiatric Association; 2013.

## *DSM-5* Diagnostic Criteria for ADHD

Box 2.5 lists *DSM-5 diagnostic criteria for ADHD*. Several criteria are noteworthy. Symptoms need to

- Have persisted for at least 6 months
- Negatively affect directly on social and academic functioning
- Present in 2 or more settings and
- Interfere with, or reduce the quality of, social, academic, or occupational functioning

Presence of 6 or more inattentive symptoms that meet the above criteria supports a diagnosis of ADHD, inattentive subtype. Presence of 6 or more hyperactive/impulsive symptoms that meet the above criteria supports a

**Box 2.5. Simplified *DSM-5* Diagnostic Criteria for ADHD[a]**

| Symptom and Duration Criteria |
| --- |
| A. A persistent pattern of inattention, hyperactivity, or both that interferes with functioning or development and is characterized by (1), (2), or both |
|    1. Inattention |
|       • Six or more inattention symptoms (see Box 2.1). |
|       • Symptoms have persisted for at least 6 months. |
|       • Degree is inconsistent with developmental level. |
|       • Negatively directly affects social and academic functioning. |
|    2. Hyperactivity and Impulsivity |
|       • Six or more hyperactivity-impulsivity symptoms (see Box 2.4). |
|       • Symptoms have persisted for at least 6 months. |
|       • Degree is inconsistent with developmental level. |
|       • Negatively directly affects social and academic functioning. |
| **Onset, Setting, and Quality of Functioning Criteria** |
| B. Several inattentive or hyperactive-impulsive symptoms were present prior to age 12 years. |
| C. Several inattentive or hyperactive-impulsive symptoms are present in 2 or more settings (eg, at home or school, with friends or relatives, in other activities). |
| D. There is clear evidence that the symptoms interfere with, or reduce quality of, social, academic, or occupational functioning. |
| **Exclusion Criteria** |
| E. Symptoms do not occur exclusively during the course of schizophrenia or another psychotic disorder and are not better explained by another mental disorder. |

Abbreviation: *DSM-5, Diagnostic and Statistical Manual of Mental Disorders, Fifth Edition.*

[a] For the full *DSM-5* diagnostic criteria, see Appendix F.

Adapted, with permission, from American Psychiatric Association. *Diagnostic and Statistical Manual of Mental Disorders.* 5th ed. Arlington, VA: American Psychiatric Association; 2013.

diagnosis of ADHD, hyperactive/impulsive subtype. Presence of 6 or more symptoms in both groups that meet the above criteria supports a diagnosis of ADHD, combined subtype.

The risk of under-diagnosis (thus not starting treatment) is the negative effect of ongoing symptoms on functioning and development. The risks of over-diagnosis include the potential stigma associated with diagnosis and the potential adverse effects of treatment. Reevaluation at regular intervals can greatly reduce these risks.

Fortunately, treatment of ADHD is rarely an emergency. Time can be taken to explore issues related to anxiety, trauma, learning problems, and substance use that can co-occur or cause similar symptoms.

When multiple diagnoses are possible, families and pediatric PCCs may be able to choose together the order in which they are explored or treated.

## Anxiety Disorders

The core symptoms of anxiety disorders are fears or phobias, worries, and somatic concerns. A common response to these symptoms among patients is avoidance of situations that generate fear or worry.

Children with anxiety can present to the pediatric PCC in various ways. Children may share their worries, fears, or somatic concerns with their caregivers, who then describe them during an office visit. In other cases, a caregiver may report that a child is excessively shy or is avoiding social or other situations (eg, coming close to dogs, being alone). Sometimes, however, children keep their fears or worries to themselves and do not share them with others. Thus, a general inquiry regarding concerns, worries, and sources of discomfort may elicit previously unidentified anxiety.

Anxiety and depression also frequently co-occur, with one set of symptoms and related behaviors exacerbating the other. When 1 of the 2 conditions is suspected, it is necessary to ask about the other as well.

Box 2.6 lists the types of symptoms associated with common pediatric anxiety disorders. Fear (or phobia) is the primary symptom of SAD (fear of being alone), SoAD (fear of embarrassment or discomfort in social situations), and specific phobia (fear of a specific stimulus [eg, heights, snakes, needles]). Worry is the primary symptom of generalized anxiety disorder (GAD) and may be focused on a wide range of topics, such as homework or friendships. Somatic concerns can occur with any anxiety disorder and may be the presenting concern at an office visit. Table 2.2 lists the reported frequency of common somatic concerns seen in pediatric anxiety disorders.[5] Avoidance is considered a secondary symptom. Common examples include avoiding social situations or phobic stimuli.

Box 2.7 lists *DSM-5* diagnostic criteria for SAD, SoAD, and GAD. All have core symptom and duration criteria, all have additional diagnosis-specific diagnostic criteria, and all require clinically significant distress or impairment in social, academic and occupational, or other important areas of functioning.

**Box 2.6. Types of Symptoms in Common Pediatric Anxiety Disorders[a]**

| Disorders With Fear or Phobia as Primary Symptom |
|---|
| • Separation anxiety disorder<br>• Social anxiety disorder<br>• Specific phobia |
| Disorders With Worry as Primary Symptom |
| Generalized anxiety disorder |
| Symptoms That May Be Present in Any Anxiety Disorder |
| • Somatic concerns<br>• Avoidance |

[a] In the *Diagnostic and Statistical Manual of Mental Disorders, Fifth Edition,* obsessive-compulsive disorder and posttraumatic stress disorder are not anxiety disorders.

**Table 2.2. Ten Most Common Somatic Symptoms in Pediatric Anxiety Disorders[a]**

| Symptom | Percent, % | Sex or Age Differences ($P < .01$) |
|---|---|---|
| Restlessness | 74 | NA |
| Feeling sick to stomach | 70 | Less common in girls |
| Blushing | 51 | NA |
| Palpitations | 48 | NA |
| Muscle tension | 45 | NA |
| Sweating | 45 | More common in 12- to 17-year-olds |
| Trembling and shaking | 43 | More common in 12- to 17-year-olds |
| Easily fatigued | 35 | NA |
| Feeling paralyzed | 32 | NA |
| Chills and hot flashes | 31 | NA |

Abbreviation: NA, not applicable.

[a] Patients studied (N = 128) were girls (n = 63) and boys (n = 65) aged 6–11 years (n = 86) and 12–17 years (n = 42).

Data were derived from Ginsburg GS, Riddle MA, Davies M. Somatic symptoms in children and adolescents with anxiety disorders. *J Am Acad Child Adolesc Psychiatry.* 2006;45(10):1179–1187 and The Research Units on Pediatric Psychopharmacology Anxiety Study Group. The Pediatric Anxiety Rating Scale (PARS): development and psychometric properties. *J Am Acad Child Adolesc Psychiatry.* 2002;41(9):1061–1069.

**Box 2.7.** *DSM-5* **Diagnostic Criteria for Common Anxiety Disorders**[a]

| Core Symptoms |
| --- |

*Separation:* Developmentally inappropriate and excessive fear or anxiety concerning separation from those to whom the youngster is attached as manifested by >3 of 8 symptoms.

*Social:* Marked fear or anxiety about >1 social situation in which the individual is exposed to possible scrutiny by others (adults or peers).

*Generalized:* Excessive anxiety and worry (apprehensive expectation), occurring more days than not, about a number of events or activities.

| Additional Disorder-Specific Diagnostic Criteria |
| --- |

*Separation:* Refer to Appendix F for a list of 8 ways in which core separation symptoms can manifest; as noted above, 3 or more are required.

*Social*
- Fears will act in a way or show anxiety symptoms that will be negatively evaluated.
- Social situations almost always provoke fear or anxiety.
- Social situations are avoided or endured with intense fear or anxiety.
- Fear or anxiety are out of proportion to actual threat posed by the social situation.

*Generalized*
- Youngster finds it difficult to control worry.
- Anxiety and worry are associated with 1 or more of 6 somatic symptoms: restless, keyed up, or on edge; easily fatigued; difficulty concentrating or mind goes blank; irritability; muscle tension; sleep disturbance.

| Impairment/Distress |
| --- |

*All 3:* Symptoms cause clinically significant distress or impairment in social, academic, occupational, or other important areas of functioning.

| Duration |
| --- |

*Separation:* Rarely presents clinically with <6 months' duration, but criterion is >4 weeks.

*Social:* 6 months.

*Generalized:* 6 months.

| Exclusions |
| --- |

*All 3:* Physiologic effects of a substance(s), another medical condition (eg, hyperthyroidism), or another mental disorder.

Abbreviation: *DSM-5, Diagnostic and Statistical Manual of Mental Disorders, Fifth Edition.*

[a] For the full *DSM-5* diagnostic criteria, see Appendix F.

Classified using American Psychiatric Association. *Diagnostic and Statistical Manual of Mental Disorders.* 5th ed. Arlington, VA: American Psychiatric Association; 2013.

The SCARED provides information about the symptoms of all common anxiety disorders as well as severity of each symptom. Parent and child versions are available (see Appendix A). Review and discussion of the SCARED symptom ratings with the child and caregiver together may be educational and can clarify difference in understanding of what is or is not a symptom and what distress and impairment may be associated with various symptoms.

Although establishing a specific diagnosis is important for helping the patient and family understand formulation and feedback, the treatment approach for all common anxiety disorders (SAD, SoAD, GAD), and simple phobias and panic attacks, is basically the same: CBT and, sometimes, medication. The specific technique a CBT therapist uses may vary by specific diagnosis, but the basic strategy is the same.

Differential diagnosis should include consideration of other medical, developmental, and mental health conditions. Repetitive or rigid behavior that may be seen in obsessive-compulsive disorder may also be present in children with autism spectrum disorder. A communication disorder may better explain failure to speak in specific social situations rather than SAD or selective mutism. Reminders of traumatic events in a child with PTSD may mimic the symptoms of GAD. Anxiety symptoms and panic attacks may occur in response to ingestion of some substances, such as methamphetamine, cocaine, or an inhalant. Certain medications, such as some decongestants, may lead to agitation, and rarely medical conditions, such as hyperthyroidism, may lead to nervousness or excessive worry, although usually other physical signs and symptoms are present as well. Also, as noted above, multiple anxiety disorders may co-occur in an individual child or adolescent.

## *Major Depressive Disorder*

### General Inquiry

The evaluation of depression in a child or adolescent may be more complex and nuanced than the evaluation of ADHD or anxiety. Many of the core symptoms of depression involve emotions and thoughts that youth can keep private. The child or adolescent, and caregiver(s), may view a clinical episode of depression as a "normal phase of growing up," or a normal effect of the angst and turmoil associated with stress, loss, interpersonal difficulties, or a variety of other problems that are common life challenges. Shame or concerns about stigma may impede their help seeking or disclosure of symptoms of depression.

Although it is important to gather information about the symptoms and diagnostic criteria of depression, it may be more productive to start with general inquiries about areas of function—school, home, family, friends, activities, and enjoyable activities. Anger and irritability may be more notice-able and important to the patient and caregiver than "depression." Talking about quality of sleep, appetite, energy, or interest in and pleasure from activities is usually easier than talking about upsetting thoughts. Once a clinical conversation is established, it is easier to progress to potentially more difficult inquiries about negative cognitions and suicidality.

## *DSM-5* Symptoms and Diagnostic Criteria

The 9 symptoms of major depressive disorder (MDD) in *DSM-5* are organized into 3 domains: mood, neurovegetative, and cognitive (Box 2.8). In children and adolescents with MDD, depressed mood usually occurs alone or in combination with irritability; rarely, irritability is the only mood symptom. Three of the 5 neurovegetative symptoms may present in the following ways: appetite and weight may be increased or decreased, sleep may be increased or decreased, and there may be psychomotor agitation or retardation.

Criterion A in the *DSM-5* diagnostic criteria (see Box 2.9) is quite specific and detailed. The episode must include all of the following:

- Five or more of the 9 symptoms in Box 2.8 must be present during the same 2-week period and must represent change from previous functioning.

**Box 2.8. *DSM-5* Symptoms of Major Depression Organized by Major Domains[a]**

| Mood |
|---|
| Depressed or irritable |
| **Neurovegetative** |
| • Weight loss or gain >5% in a month<br>• Insomnia or hypersomnia<br>• Psychomotor agitation or retardation<br>• Fatigue or loss of energy<br>• Diminished interest or pleasure |
| **Cognitive** |
| • Decreased concentration or indecisiveness<br>• Worthlessness or guilt<br>• Suicidal ideation |

Abbreviation: *DSM-5*, *Diagnostic and Statistical Manual of Mental Disorders, Fifth Edition.*

[a] For the full *DSM-5* diagnostic criteria, see Appendix F.

Classified using American Psychiatric Association. *Diagnostic and Statistical Manual of Mental Disorders.* 5th ed. Arlington, VA: American Psychiatric Association; 2013.

**Box 2.9. Simplified *DSM-5* Diagnostic Criteria for Major Depressive Disorder[a]**

A. Episode must include
  - Five or more of the 9 symptoms in Box 2.8
  - Symptoms that present during the same 2-week period
  - Symptoms that represent change from previous functioning
  - Symptoms that present nearly every day (except weight change and suicidal ideation)
  - At least one symptom that is depressed or irritable mood or loss of interest or pleasure

B. Symptoms cause clinically significant distress or impairment in social, occupational, or other important areas of functioning.

C. Episode is not attributable to the physiologic effects of a substance or to another medical condition.

D. Episode is not better explained by another major psychiatric disorder, such as a psychotic disorder.

E. There has never been a manic episode or a hypomanic episode.

Abbreviation: *DSM-5, Diagnostic and Statistical Manual of Mental Disorders, Fifth Edition.*

[a] For the full *DSM-5* diagnostic criteria, see Appendix F.

Classified using American Psychiatric Association. *Diagnostic and Statistical Manual of Mental Disorders.* 5th ed. Arlington, VA: American Psychiatric Association; 2013.

- Symptoms must be present nearly every day (except weight change and suicidal ideation).
- At least one of the symptoms must be depressed or irritable mood or loss of interest or pleasure.
- In addition, the symptoms must cause clinically significant distress or impairment in social, occupational, or other important areas of functioning.
- Taken together, these diagnostic criteria make it clear that an episode of MDD is a discrete and relatively specific clinical entity.

Although the minimum duration requirement for an episode of depression is just 2 weeks, children or adolescents may present with symptoms that have been present for many weeks or even months. Such a chronic presentation can make it more challenging to accurately delineate a discrete episode of depression.

## Recovery From an Episode

Recovery from an episode of depression often starts with improvement in neurovegetative symptoms, such as sleep, appetite, and energy. Improvement in cognitive symptoms—feelings of worthlessness or guilt and suicidal ideation—usually occurs later. The period between improvement of neurovegetative symptoms and improvement of cognitive symptoms is considered a period of high risk for suicide attempts because the patient may have more energy and vitality to act on lingering suicidal thoughts.

## Rating Scales

The PHQ-9 Modified for Teens and *Guidelines for the Management of Adolescent Depression in Primary Care (GLAD-PC)* (see Appendix A) may be helpful in eliciting symptoms of depression. However, there is no available shortcut to the accurate diagnosis of an episode of MDD.

## Differential Diagnosis

Differential diagnosis of MDD in youth can be a challenge. Children who are demoralized by various family, social, medical, peer, academic, or other problems can exhibit many of the symptoms of MDD. Demoralized children often have mood and cognitive symptoms identical to those in children with MDD, but neurovegetative symptoms are less likely to be present. Grief can also mimic MDD. The prominent affect in grief is feelings of emptiness or loss, in contrast with depressed mood or the inability to anticipate happiness or pleasure in MDD. Trauma- and stress-related disorders, such as adjustment disorder with depressed mood, may also mimic MDD. The essential distinguishing feature of adjustment disorder is an identifiable stressor that precedes the mood symptoms.

## Safety Assessment and Monitoring

An important part of the evaluation and treatment of MDD is a safety assessment. Safety of the home needs to be reviewed, including access to weapons, potentially lethal medications, and other objects and substances that could facilitate a suicide attempt.

The parents' ability to monitor the patient needs to be carefully evaluated; suicide attempts almost always occur when the child is not being monitored. Evaluation of the patient needs to include inquires such as, "What would you do if you had thoughts or urges to make a suicide attempt? Whom would you inform of such thoughts or urges?" A child's inability or unwillingness to provide reassuring responses to these questions may indicate that it is not safe to send the child home.

## Extended Evaluations and Interim Check-ins

It is not always possible to complete an initial evaluation of depression that results in sufficient enough clarity regarding diagnosis and safety to facilitate a coherent treatment plan. In such situations, it is useful to schedule a follow-up evaluation appointment relatively soon and, in the interim, to conduct brief phone check-ins with the parents and the patient. Check-ins should include review of symptoms, functioning, monitoring, and safety. Even if a referral to a child and adolescent psychiatrist or other specialist is initiated at the first evaluation visit, interim check-ins should be done until the time of the child's first specialist appointment.

## Assessment of Common Comorbidities

Attention-deficit/hyperactivity disorder, anxiety, and depression often co-occur. Thus, assessment of each of these 3 common disorders is recommended, even when the presenting concern or the results of initial screening indicates that 1 of the 3 is prominent. The presence of other comorbidities typically suggests the need for specialty consultation and comanagement. These include the following disorders.

### Disruptive Behavioral Problems and Disorders

Disruptive behaviors, except for severe aggression and major antisocial acts, rarely occur without the presence of other mental health conditions. Disorders such as ADHD, depression, other mood disorders, and adjustment disorders are usually present in a child or adolescent with disruptive behavior. In addition, children with disruptive behaviors often receive negative attention from caregivers, siblings, peers, and others; the result is a feedback loop that unintentionally reinforces and sustains the disruptive behaviors. Disruptive behavioral problems are common, particularly in children with ADHD. Usually these disruptive behaviors are mild to moderate in severity, although they can be quite impairing in home or school settings.

There is considerable controversy about the appropriateness and validity of "pure" disruptive behavioral diagnoses. *Diagnostic and Statistical Manual of Mental Disorders, Fourth Edition* (*DSM-IV*) included a diagnosis that was commonly used to codify mild-to-moderate disruptive behaviors: *disruptive behavior disorder not otherwise specified* (NOS). In *DSM-5*, disruptive behavior disorder NOS was eliminated and replaced with 2 diagnostic options that can be used for youth with mild-to-moderate disruptive behaviors: *other specified disruptive, impulse-control, and conduct disorder* and *unspecified disruptive, impulse-control, and conduct disorder*. The former (*other*) is used when a specific reason for not meeting diagnostic criteria can be or is provided; the latter (*unspecified*) is used when a specific reason cannot be or is not provided. The names of these diagnoses are long and cumbersome. More problematic is that these "default" diagnoses provide no specific diagnostic criteria appropriate to children. Further, they are the default diagnoses for conduct disorder and intermittent explosive disorder, which are severe, rare in children, and relatively uncommon in adolescents. For more information on the assessment and treatment of aggression, refer to T-MAY (see Appendix A).

## Behavioral and Mood Disorders

*Oppositional defiant disorder* (ODD) has a pejorative name that highlights "bad" behavior. However, ODD has 3 domains: angry or irritable mood (3 symptoms), argumentative or defiant behavior (4 symptoms), and vindictiveness (1 symptom). At least 4 symptoms lasting at least 6 months are required to meet diagnostic criteria. A diagnosis of ODD can be useful in helping parents and caregivers understand this pattern of negative behavior that can result in significant parenting stress. The Vanderbilt Assessment Scale for ADHD (see Appendix A) includes items that can serve as a screener for ODD, which occurs commonly in children with ADHD.

In an extreme example of primarily mood symptoms, a child could receive a diagnosis of ODD by having 3 mood symptoms and only one behavioral symptom, such as "*often* blames others for his or her mistakes or behaviors." At the other extreme, a child could receive a diagnosis of ODD with 4 behavioral symptoms and no mood symptoms. The symptoms and diagnostic criteria for ODD are presented in Boxes 2.10 and 2.11.

The estimated prevalence of ODD is about 3%, indicating that it is a common disorder.[6] Of note, symptom severity in children with ODD is reduced considerably in response to treatment of comorbid disorders, particularly ADHD.[7] Behavioral management training for parents is often effective.

*Disruptive mood dysregulation disorder* (DMDD) is a new diagnosis in *DSM-5* (see Box 2.12). Before *DSM-5*, there was considerable controversy about how to diagnose bipolar disorder in children and adolescents who did not meet criteria for bipolar disorder but did have mood instability or irritability and behavioral outbursts. Mood disorder NOS became the default diagnosis for these youth. At the same time, there was concern about excessive and inappropriate diagnosis of bipolar disorder in youth, especially preteens. Subsequent research identified a group of children and adolescents with chronic irritability and intermittent disruptive behaviors. The proposed label for this group was severe mood dysregulation.[8,9] Disruptive mood dysregulation disorder is based, largely, on research about severe mood dysregulation.

### Box 2.10. Simplified *DSM-5* Symptoms of Oppositional Defiant Disorder[a,b]

| Angry or Irritable Mood |
|---|
| • Loses temper<br>• Touchy or easily annoyed<br>• Angry and resentful |
| **Argumentative or Defiant Behavior** |
| • Argues with adults<br>• Actively defies or refuses to comply with requests from authority figures or with rules<br>• Deliberately annoys others<br>• Blames others for his or her mistakes or misbehavior |
| **Vindictiveness** |
| Spiteful or vindictive |

Abbreviation: *DSM-5, Diagnostic and Statistical Manual of Mental Disorders, Fifth Edition.*

[a] Frequency of symptoms must be *often*, except for vindictiveness, which is at least twice within the past 6 months.

[b] For the full *DSM-5* diagnostic criteria, see Appendix F.

Classified using American Psychiatric Association. *Diagnostic and Statistical Manual of Mental Disorders.* 5th ed. Arlington, VA: American Psychiatric Association; 2013.


### Box 2.11. Simplified *DSM-5* Diagnostic Criteria for Oppositional Defiant Disorder[a]

| Symptom and Duration Criteria[b] |
|---|
| • Persistent pattern of angry or irritable mood, argumentative or defiant behavior, or vindictiveness<br>• Lasting at least 6 months<br>• With at least 4 symptoms from Box 2.10<br>• Exhibited during interaction with at least one individual who is not a sibling |
| **Functional Impairment Criteria** |
| • Distress in the child or others in his or her immediate social context (eg, family, peer group, fellow students)<br>• Negatively affects social, educational, or other important areas of functioning |
| **Exclusion Criteria** |
| • Behaviors do not occur exclusively during the course of a psychotic, substance use, depressive, or bipolar disorder.<br>• Criteria are not met for disruptive mood dysregulation disorder. |
| **Severity** |
| • *Mild:* Symptoms confined to only one setting (eg, at home, at school, with peers).<br>• *Moderate:* Symptoms present in at least 2 settings.<br>• *Severe:* Symptoms present in 3 or more settings. |

Abbreviation: *DSM-5, Diagnostic and Statistical Manual of Mental Disorders, Fifth Edition.*

[a] For the full *DSM-5* diagnostic criteria, see Appendix F.

[b] Persistence and frequency of these behaviors should be used to distinguish a behavior that is within normal limits from a behavior that is symptomatic. For children younger than 5 years, the behavior should occur on most days for a period of at least 6 months, except for vindictiveness. For children 5 years or older, the behavior should occur at least once per week for at least 6 months, except for vindictiveness.

Classified using American Psychiatric Association. *Diagnostic and Statistical Manual of Mental Disorders.* 5th ed. Arlington, VA: American Psychiatric Association; 2013.

The core features of DMDD are chronic, severe, and persistent irritability and frequent temper outbursts. The outbursts can be verbal or physical (or both), including aggression against property or individuals. The chronicity of irritability is what differentiates DMDD from ODD, MDD, or bipolar disorder, all of which can include irritability that is episodic or periodic but not chronic.

Because DMDD is new and has not been studied extensively, prevalence estimates are speculative but are probably in the 2% to 5% range among children and adolescents.[6] Children and adolescents with DMDD are at risk to develop depression or anxiety disorders (or both) in adulthood. Risk of later development of bipolar disorder is small. Because *DSM-5* first appeared in 2013, research on evidence-based treatments is not widely available.

## Other Comorbid Disorders

*Adjustment disorders* with depressed mood, anxiety, disturbance of conduct, or any combination of these 3 symptoms are common in children and adolescents. The core feature of an adjustment disorder is the development of clinically significant emotional or behavioral symptoms within 3 months of an identifiable stressor. Of note, a recent identifiable stressor does not preclude another diagnosis instead of or in addition to an adjustment disorder (eg, ADHD, an anxiety disorder, MDD, ODD, DMDD). Adjustment disorders are common, although prevalence estimates are inconsistent.

*Substance use disorders* are common in adolescents. As noted previously, for preteens and adolescents, screening for substance use is recommended. The CRAFFT substance abuse screening questionnaire is a validated, brief pediatric screening tool (www.ceasar-boston.org/clinicians/crafft.php).

Successful assessment and treatment of any psychiatric disorder is difficult, if not impossible, if there is significant ongoing substance abuse. These situations may require referral to a substance abuse specialist or program. Minimal substance use may not require specialty referral.

Estimated 12-month prevalence of alcohol use disorder is about 5% in 12- to 17-year-olds.[6] Estimated 12-month prevalence of cannabis use disorder is 3.4% in 12- to 17-year-olds.[6] Prevalence of use disorders for other drugs in adolescents is much lower.

*Learning disabilities or disorders, mild intellectual disability (ID), and communication disorders* are likely to be suspected or diagnosed during well-child visits or by caregivers or school personnel. Confirmation of these conditions

**Box 2.12. Simplified *DSM-5* Diagnostic Criteria for Disruptive Mood Dysregulation Disorder[a]**

| Symptom Criteria |
| --- |

Severe recurrent temper outbursts
- Manifested verbally (eg, verbal rages), behaviorally (eg, physical aggression toward people or property), or both
- Grossly out of proportion in intensity or duration to the situation or provocation

Temper outbursts
- Are inconsistent with developmental level
- Occur, on average, 3 or more times per week

Mood between temper outbursts
- Persistently irritable or angry
- Most of the day
- Nearly every day
- Observable by others (eg, parents, teachers, peers)

| Duration, Setting, and Onset Criteria |
| --- |

Symptom criteria (above) have been present
- Twelve or more months
- Without a period of ≥3 consecutive months without symptom criteria met

Symptom criteria are
- Present in at least 2 of 3 settings (ie, at home, at school, with peers)
- Severe in at least 1 of these settings

Diagnosis should *not* be made
- First time before age 6 years or
- After age 18 years

Age of onset is before 10 years by history or observation.

| Exclusion Criteria |
| --- |

- Manic or hypomanic episode
- Not exclusively during major depressive episode
- Not better explained by another mental disorder
- Not attributable to substances or medical or neurologic conditions

Abbreviation: *DSM-5, Diagnostic and Statistical Manual of Mental Disorders, Fifth Edition.*

[a] For the full *DSM-5* diagnostic criteria, see Appendix F.

Adapted, with permission, from American Psychiatric Association. *Diagnostic and Statistical Manual of Mental Disorders.* 5th ed. Arlington, VA: American Psychiatric Association; 2013.

requires formal testing, which is usually provided by the child's school system. For the further evaluation of a child with suspected learning disability or disorder, ID, or a communication disorder, consultation and collaboration with specialists in neurodevelopmental disorders is recommended. The prevalence of specific learning disorders across the academic domains of reading, writing, and mathematics ranges from 5% to 15%.[6] The prevalence of ID is about 1%.[6]

*Sleep disorders* include insomnia, sleep apnea, narcolepsy, and restless legs syndrome. Insomnia is the most common pediatric sleep disorder. The core symptom of insomnia is an inability to fall or stay asleep that can result in functional impairment throughout the day (www.cdc.gov/features/sleep). Insomnia cannot be attributable to the physiologic effects of a substance or coexisting mental disorders or medical conditions. Thus, a primary diagnosis of insomnia is usually made if sleep disruption continues after treatment of medical and mental disorders. Consultation with a pediatric sleep specialist is recommended when primary insomnia is suspected.

## Assessment of Less Common Comorbidities

Less common disorders, which have a prevalence in children and adolescents of less than about 1%, are usually severe and quite impairing and can be recognized, or at least suspected, because of unique characteristic symptoms. Some of these less common disorders and characteristic symptoms are

- Autism spectrum disorder: social communication deficits and restricted repetitive behaviors or interests
- Schizophrenia: hallucinations, delusions, disordered thinking
- Bipolar: manic episodes
- Eating: weight loss, food restriction, binging, purging
- Conduct: behavior violating others' rights and social norms
- Posttraumatic stress: intrusive memories, dissociative experiences, and avoidance or arousal symptoms in response to exposure to actual or threatened death, serious injury, or sexual violation
- Obsessive-compulsive: obsessions or compulsions (or both)

If these or similar comorbidities are suspected, referral to a specialist for a full evaluation and treatment is recommended.

# Formulation and Feedback

Formulation and feedback for children and adolescents with mental disorders and their caregivers and families requires skill and practice. The trusting and often longitudinal relationship between pediatric PCCs and their patients is an important factor in reducing the stress and discomfort that families often experience when discussing these types of sensitive topics. Key points in the feedback process are presented on the next page.

## Emphasize Positive Attributes

The pediatric PCC can strengthen engagement with the caregiver(s) and child by reviewing positive attributes of the child and family and highlighting these as protective factors for the child. It is worth noting that both short- and long-term outcome are greatly influenced by positive attributes.

## Review Key Points of the History

A brief review of the history can be helpful in allowing the family to feel heard and that the PCC has "gotten it right" before embarking on a diagnosis and subsequent treatment plan. This can also help reduce resistance going forward as potentially sensitive diagnoses or interventions are discussed.

## Normalize the Feedback Experience

Families should be aware that mental health problems are common in children and are not the result of character flaws or bad parenting. If medication is being considered, presenting the disorder as similar to other medical illnesses (eg, asthma, strep throat) that respond well to medication helps normalize the feedback experience and minimize blame and guilt.

If there is another family member(s) who has the same diagnosis as the identified child, and particularly if this family member has responded well to treatment, reviewing his or her experience can help normalize the diagnosis and offer real hope regarding outcome. Conversely, if a family member has not responded well to treatment, it may be helpful to differentiate that family member's experience from the present circumstances.

Several things cannot be said too often: common disorders are common, many children and adolescents have them, most do well, and the prognosis, especially for ADHD, anxiety, and depression, is generally positive.

## Develop a Basic Formulation

Formulating involves synthesizing and integrating various factors precipitating and perpetuating a disorder(s) and promoting a successful intervention. Communicating a basic formulation includes

- Emphasizing positive attributes of the patient and family
- Instilling confidence that the presenting concerns can be effectively treated
- Describing and inviting discussion of diagnostic impressions and the evidence the clinician has used to arrive at those impressions

- Listing possible diagnoses that require further evaluation, or other steps in evaluation, that could be taken if the family desires or if the working impression does not lead to successful treatment
- When indicated, mentioning that other possible attributes (aka "perspectives")[10] may be contributing to the illness and may be factors in choosing among possible treatments, including
  - Personality traits (eg, introversion)
  - Intellectual and learning strengths and weaknesses
  - Behaviors that may need immediate attention (eg, suicide attempts)
  - The effect of experiences in the family, with peers, and in school
  - The child's internalization and integration of those experiences

The "possible attributes" noted above may need to be explored by a specialist. They are also generally in the domain of child psychiatrists, psychologists, and other mental health specialists in both evaluation and treatment. These other attributes are not features of a mental disorder or illness and are not treatable with medication. They may be responsive to various psychotherapies.

## Prioritize Problems and Diagnoses

If more than one problem or diagnosis will benefit from treatment, it is important to discuss which should be addressed first and why. Prioritization is an ongoing and collaborative process and may change over time depending on the patient's response to the initial treatment plan. Thus, treatment targets may need to be updated over time.

## Discuss Prognosis

For most children, and for most common disorders, it is possible to be positive about prognosis, if treatment is implemented. Response to short-term treatment can improve the validity of long-term prognostication. Reiterating one's long-term commitment to the patient and caregiver(s) may also improve the long-term outlook of the patient and caregiver(s).

## Emphasize the High Rate of Success of Available Treatments

Emphasize that evidence-based treatments, both medication and psychotherapy, are highly effective. Most patients who adhere to treatment improve substantially. Defining goals that are important to the child and family will also help improve engagement and treatment. Similarly, when several treatment options are present, presenting a brief "menu of options" can allow for individualized treatment plans tailored to the needs and preferences of the family.

## Clarify Plans for Referral and Communicate With Other Professionals

The need for additional evaluation, whether by the pediatric PCC or a specialist, or both, needs to be noted and explained. Knowing that other professionals will be involved in the evaluation process (and treatment) may be reassuring to the family.

Patient and caregiver(s) will want to know who will be in the circle of communication (eg, school personnel, mental health specialists, other family members). It is important to describe the nature of the communications and confidentiality and to address any concerns.

## Approach Evaluation as a Continuously Evolving Process

Because most mental disorders are chronic and are affected by ongoing development and life experiences, evaluation is a continuously evolving process. It is likely that follow-up evaluations will be shorter and simpler than the initial evaluation but are not less important.

# References

1. Foy JM; American Academy of Pediatrics Task Force on Mental Health. Enhancing pediatric mental health care: algorithms for primary care. *Pediatrics.* 2010;125 (Suppl 3):S109–S125
2. Hertzman C, Boyce T. How experience gets under the skin to create gradients in developmental health. *Ann Rev Public Health.* 2010;31:329–347
3. Wissow L, Anthony B, Brown J, et al. A common factors approach to improving the mental health capacity of pediatric primary care. *Adm Policy Ment Health.* 2008;35(4): 305–318
4. Wolraich M, Brown RT, DuPaul G, et al; American Academy of Pediatrics Subcommittee on Attention-Deficit/Hyperactivity Disorder; Steering Committee on Quality Improvement. ADHD: clinical practice guideline for the diagnosis, evaluation, and treatment of attention-deficit/hyperactivity disorder in children and adolescents. *Pediatrics.* 2011;128(5):1007–1022
5. Ginsburg GS, Riddle MA, Davies M. Somatic symptoms in children and adolescents with anxiety disorders. *J Am Acad Child Adolesc Psychiatry.* 2006;45(10):1179–1187
6. American Psychiatric Association. *Diagnostic and Statistical Manual of Mental Disorders.* 5th ed. Arlington, VA: American Psychiatric Association; 2013
7. The MTA Cooperative Group. A 14-month randomized clinical trial of treatment strategies for attention-deficit/hyperactivity disorder: multimodal treatment study of children with ADHD. *Arch Gen Psychiatry.* 1999;56(12):1073–1086
8. Leibenluft E, Charney DS, Towbin KE, Bhangoo RK, Pine DS. Defining clinical phenotypes of juvenile mania. *Am J Psychiatry.* 2003;160(3):430–437

9. Leibenluft E. Severe mood dysregulation, irritability, and the diagnostic boundaries of bipolar disorder in youths. *Am J Psychiatry.* 2011;168(2):129–142

10. McHugh PR, Slavney PR. *The Perspectives of Psychiatry.* 2nd ed. Baltimore, MD: Johns Hopkins University Press; 1998

# CHAPTER 3

# Prescribing Medications: Getting Started

This chapter presents practical guidance for pediatric primary care clinicians (pediatric PCCs) regarding safe and effective prescribing and monitoring of psychotropic medications. We will look at some of the key factors that will aid in effective treatment.

## Conditions for Safe and Effective Prescribing

Safe and effective use of psychotropic medications in the primary care setting depends on meeting several important conditions across several domains. These domains are

- Disorder
- Medication
- Dosing and monitoring parameters
- Capacity and comfort of the prescribing pediatric PCC
- System of care

Box 3.1 provides an "ideal" list of such conditions. Obviously, not all can be met in all settings (eg, adequate financial reimbursement).

## Non-medication Treatments

Treatment interventions can be of several types.

- Clinical leadership
- Guidance
- Pragmatic supports
- Evidence-based psychotherapy
- Medication

**Box 3.1. Conditions for Safe and Effective Prescribing of Psychotropic Medications by Pediatric Primary Care Clinicians**

| |
|---|
| The *disorder* for which medication is prescribed needs to be<br>• Sufficiently common to be seen regularly by a pediatric PCC<br>• Efficiently and accurately diagnosable by a pediatric PCC |
| The *medication* needs to<br>• Have demonstrated efficacy<br>• Be relatively safe, as assessed by several parameters<br>• Have adverse effects that are reasonably predictable, readily detected, and readily managed |
| The *dosing and monitoring* of the medication need to<br>• Follow guidelines that are reasonably established and easily followed<br>• Include somatic monitoring that is limited to vital signs and height and weight |
| The *prescribing physician* needs to have<br>• Expertise in diagnosing relevant disorders<br>• Knowledge of available psychosocial treatments (eg, PBMT, CBT)<br>• Knowledge of medications prescribed<br>• Procedures for monitoring medication effects and adherence |
| The *system of care* needs to provide<br>• Access to pediatric psychopharmacology expertise for consultation on issues beyond the expertise of the pediatric PCC<br>• Adequate payment for services rendered<br>• Minimal administrative and regulatory barriers |

Abbreviations: CBT, cognitive-behavioral therapy; PBMT, parent behavioral management training; PCC, primary care clinician.

## Clinical Leadership

Pediatric PCCs are familiar with, and experts at, providing various types of clinical leadership, including

- Coordinating care
- Collaborating with colleagues
- Obtaining consultations
- Referring
- Providing support
- Accessing resources

Although often underappreciated and rarely adequately reimbursed, clinical leadership is the bedrock of an effective treatment plan. When more than one clinician is involved in the mental health care of a patient, someone needs to assure that care is coordinated and that communication between the clinicians, caregiver, patient, school, and relevant others is conducted consistently and effectively. The pediatric PCC is usually best suited to play this role.

## Guidance

Pediatric PCCs are accustomed to offering youth and caregivers guidance in managing interpersonal and behavioral problems. They can apply "common factors" communication techniques (so-called because they are derived from evidence-based approaches effective across multiple conditions) to engage patients and families in problem-solving. These techniques may be applicable, for example, to poor sleep hygiene, sibling conflict, stress management, adolescent "rebellion," and unhealthy habits, such as excessive use of social media. In addition, pediatric PCCs can apply these techniques to engaging caregivers in addressing their own issues that affect their child's well-being (eg, maternal depression, marital discord, and substance abuse). See Appendix C.

## Pragmatic Supports

Pragmatic supports are social, economic, and academic resources that enhance the ability of the overall treatment plan to succeed. Examples include academic tutoring, parent-to-parent support groups, funds for transportation to psychotherapy sessions, and assistance in addressing other environmental and socioeconomic issues that influence mental health, such as poor-quality child care, food insecurity, poverty, and unsafe housing. For more information on evidence-informed pragmatic supports, see Appendix C.

## Evidence-Based Psychotherapy

Evidence-based psychotherapies are administered by trained therapists who use detailed treatment manuals for regularly scheduled sessions (usually weekly) over 8 to 12 weeks or longer. The most relevant and commonly prescribed evidence-based psychotherapies for the common pediatric disorders (attention-deficit/hyperactivity disorder [ADHD], anxiety, and depression) are behavioral management training (BMT) for parents or caregivers and cognitive behavioral therapy (CBT) for the child or adolescent.

In general, psychotherapies are labor- and time intensive. They require specific training and availability of the therapist, as well as a commitment from the child's parent or caregiver. An extensive listing of virtually all known psychotherapies for youth is provided by PracticeWise to the American Academy of Pediatrics (AAP) (www.aap.org/mentalhealth) and is updated at regular intervals; it does not reflect AAP policy. (See Appendix D.) For clinical practice purposes, the Level 1—BEST SUPPORT column is most relevant. It is important to be aware of the therapies in Level 4—MINIMAL SUPPORT and Level 5—NO SUPPORT because these are still commonly used and are of no or very minimal documented benefit.

Evidence from large studies sponsored by the National Institute for Mental Health demonstrates the advantage of combining psychotherapy and medication treatment over medication or therapy alone for ADHD (ages 7–9 years),[1] common anxiety disorders (separation anxiety disorder, social phobia, generalized anxiety disorder; ages 7–17),[2] and depression (ages 12–17).[3] The additional effect of combined treatment over only medication or psychotherapy is clinically meaningful, but relatively small. However, psychotherapy alone may be preferred over medication or combination treatment for initial care of mild symptoms.

It is important to consider when psychosocial interventions are preferred over medication. Many children and adolescents present to pediatric PCCs with mild depression or anxiety (ie, they meet diagnostic criteria, but symptoms and impairment are minimal) or subthreshold depression or anxiety (ie, they do not meet diagnostic criteria for the disorder but report more than minimal impairment). In general, such a child is likely to benefit from an evidence-based psychosocial intervention and may not need medication. For preschool-aged children, guidelines recommend at least 2 trials of psychosocial treatment before starting medication.[4]

Despite clear effectiveness of various psychotherapies and the pressing need for them, far too few mental health clinicians are licensed—including clinical psychologists, social workers, nurse practitioners, certified counselors, and some child and adolescent psychiatrists—with proper training and experience to provide high-quality evidence-based psychotherapy. Families also face many administrative and financial barriers to access. For many pediatric PCCs, the shortage of qualified therapists, along with occasional caregiver resistance to psychotherapy, adds pressure to prescribe psychopharmacologic therapy as a single first-line treatment.

Unfortunately, there are no quick, brief, effective, evidence-based psychotherapies designed for primary care practice that have been successfully disseminated and broadly implemented. The best currently available is the Triple P – Positive Parenting Program, which offers a brief, evidence-based intervention aimed at primary care, although dissemination has been limited.[5-7] A new evidence-informed approach, which is still under study, draws on "common elements" of evidence-based psychotherapies that are readily applied in primary care (eg, relaxation techniques and gradual exposure for anxiety, visualization techniques and behavioral activation for depression) to create initial primary care interventions for children whose conditions do not yet rise to the level of a disorder or whose families are not yet ready to seek care from a therapist. This approach is incorporated into guidance offered by the World Health Organization and adapted by the AAP in the book *Signs and Symptoms in Pediatrics*.[8]

These approaches notwithstanding, pediatric PCCs often are left feeling no alternative but to prescribe medication without psychotherapy. In such cases, an ideal time to revisit the recommendation of psychotherapy is when or if the initial medication trial is ineffective or not well tolerated.

A recent and methodologically sound study found that for ADHD being treated in community-based pediatric settings, while 93% of patients were receiving medication, only 13% were receiving non-medication treatment.[9] Pediatric PCCs can join with families and mental health specialists in their communities to advocate for evidence-based psychotherapies in both public and private systems of care. Ideally, non-medication interventions always accompany pharmacologic interventions. Information and resources about evidence-based and commonly used non-medication interventions are provided in Appendix D.

# Informed Consent

The process of obtaining informed consent from the parent or guardian and assent from the patient can be more complicated and difficult for psychotropic medications than other medications. This is because of parental concerns about the potential effect of medications on the child's developing brain and controversy in the media regarding psychotropic medications. Thus, in addition to the initial consent process, informed consent is usually an ongoing process that unfolds over time as the patient and caregiver(s) develop new questions and concerns about medication(s).

Informed consent and assent have 2 aspects: the medicolegal consent document and the clinical consent process.

For medicolegal consent documentation, there appears to be wide variation, including such practices as[10]

- Use of a specific required form that must be completed (a practice that is likely to expand with increased use of electronic records, particularly in large health care systems)
- Required written documentation without a specific required form
- No documentation of consent

The American Academy of Child and Adolescent Psychiatry "Practice Parameters on the Use of Psychotropic Medication in Children and Adolescents"[11] provides detailed information about the process of consent but is silent regarding documentation.

For clinical consent, the basic process of obtaining informed consent and assent is the same, no matter what psychotropic medication is recommended. A description of domains to cover in the consent process is provided in Table 3.1. Completing this process requires considerable time and effort and is clearly a challenge given time and reimbursement limitations in primary care. To meet this challenge, it may be useful and efficient to have a designated staff member assist the prescribing clinician with the details of consent, as is commonly done for immunizations and other prescriptions and procedures in outpatient practices.

Informed consent is not permanent but rather an ongoing and evolving discussion. An ideal time to discuss the need for ongoing reevaluation of treatment and consent is during the initial consent process. It is important to establish a timeline for reevaluating medication efficacy and adverse effects and to note that consent can and will be revisited in light of the patient's initial and ongoing responses to and experiences with the medication, both positive and negative. Thus, consent is an ongoing component of an evolving clinical process.

# Adherence and Persistence

Medications that are not ingested are not effective.[12] Unfortunately, rate of non-adherence in pediatric psychopharmacology is not well studied or documented, except for stimulants, for which data suggest high levels of non-adherence.[13] Parent reports of adherence to sustained-release stimulant preparations indicate about 10% to 25% of non-adherence. Even more

**Table 3.1. A Clinical Approach to the Process of Informed Consent for Psychotropic Medication**

**1. Preamble**
- Conceptualization of signs and symptoms as *illness*.
- What are the *risks of not treating* with medication?
- Think *job performance* (home, school, friends).
- Think *development* (emotional, behavioral, social, cognitive).

**2. Evidence Supporting Short-term Efficacy and Effectiveness**
- A level: 2 (or 1 if sufficiently worthy) placebo-controlled, random-assignment studies[a]
- B level: 1 placebo-controlled, random-assignment, properly implemented study
- C level: information from open-label studies, case reports, etc

**3. Alternative or Additional Treatments**
- Evidence-based psychotherapies
- Community, family, and school-system support
- Other medications

**4. Adverse Effects**

| Severity | Change needed | Examples |
|---|---|---|
| Mild | Requires no change | Dry mouth, transient nausea |
| Moderate | Requires dose change | Sedation |
| Severe | Requires stopping drug | Real suicidal ideation or attempt |

**5. Potential Long-term Adverse Effects**
- Examples: growth retardation (stimulants), diabetes mellitus, or tardive dyskinesia (antipsychotics)
- Unknown

**6. Pharmacokinetic Issues**
- Convenience: once-daily dosing preferred, no laboratory monitoring preferred
- Drug-drug interactions: especially involving hepatic CYP450 isoenzymes

**7. Adherence**
- Importance of establishing a convenient daily routine for taking the medication

**8. Cost**
- Generic vs brand
- Insurance coverage
- This drug vs others in class

**Bottom Line: Your Opinion About Benefit-to-Risk Ratio for This Patient**
- Taking into consideration all of the above, what do you recommend?
- Why?
- *Think: If this were your child, what would you do?*

[a] This applies to all Group 1 medications for attention-deficit/hyperactivity disorder, anxiety, and depression.

concerning, a retrospective analysis of the Multimodal Treatment Study of ADHD[1] found that only 3% of parents reported that their child did not receive prescribed stimulant medication on the day of a study visit, while child saliva samples indicated that 25% of children were non-adherent.[14] Higher levels of adherence were associated with greater improvement in ADHD symptoms. Taken together, studies of parent reports and salivary samples indicate that non-adherence to stimulant medication is an important clinical issue.

*Persistence* is the term used by epidemiologists to describe continuity of treatment. Because ADHD is a chronic disorder, relatively long-term treatment with stimulants would be expected, except during drug holidays or when stimulants are discontinued because of unacceptable adverse effects or lack of adequate therapeutic effect. However, data from community practice settings suggest that treatment is not persistent. In a study of more than 9,500 pharmacy and medical claims for 6- to 12-year-olds, Olfson and colleagues[15] found that mean duration of stimulant treatment episodes was only about 145 days for immediate-release preparations and about 150 to 160 days for longer-acting preparations. In a study using Medicaid claims for more than 40,000 5- to 20-year-olds, Winterstein and colleagues[16] found that 27% to 50% were persistent for 12 months, allowing for a 1- or 3-month gap in use, respectively. These, and other, studies suggest that most children receiving stimulants do not receive them for more than a year.

Before making decisions about dose increases, it is critically important to assess adherence. Pediatric PCCs can set the stage for this recurring assessment by providing information about adherence and non-adherence in a nonjudgmental manner before prescribing a medication. Emphasizing the importance of "tracking" medication adherence (ie, "just keep me informed about how often [Jane] did or didn't get or take her medication; then we can work together to make decisions about [Jane's] care"), rather than emphasizing actual adherence (eg, "she needs to take the medicine at least 90% of the time") can facilitate openness about medication adherence. Although not always easy, it is important to establish a therapeutic approach in which children and parents understand that assessing adherence is part of the therapeutic process and will not lead to negative judgment.

When the pediatric PCC strongly suspects non-adherence but cannot elicit confirming history, it may be necessary and useful to speak with the pharmacist who filled the prescription(s) or, when possible, review the insurance claims. While regular refills do not necessarily confirm daily adherence, their absence can, at times, provide documentation of non-adherence. Improving adherence and persistence is not a simple or easy task.[13] Specific interventions to improve adherence,[17-22] referral to a specialist, or both may be useful. Continuing to increase dose in these situations is not recommended.

# Phases of Treatment

Medication treatment for ADHD, anxiety, or depression is often initiated during an acute clinical crisis when the child's symptoms are at their worst. Thus, doses that are used in the acute phase of illness or treatment may be higher than are needed later, during subacute or maintenance treatment. This is especially true if the child and family are responsive to evidence-based psychosocial therapy that is initiated during the acute clinical crisis or shortly thereafter. Improved coping skills, more useful cognitive and behavioral constructs, reduced family tension, or successful behavioral feedback may reduce the need for medication either partially (eg, lower dose) or completely (eg, discontinuation).

On the other hand, over the longer term, doses may need to be increased in response to growth and maturation.

# Off-label Prescribing

Before the mid-1990s, very few psychotropic medications had been approved by the US Food and Drug Administration (FDA) for pediatric indications (ie, approved for use in children younger than 18 years). Those approved included stimulants for ADHD, tricyclic antidepressants for enuresis, a few antipsychotics for psychosis, and lithium for mania in bipolar disorder. Thus, to treat psychiatric disorders in children and adolescents, it was often necessary to prescribe off-label.

Although many medications still lack FDA-approved pediatric indications across the age span, the number of pediatric indications has increased markedly over the past 20 years. This has occurred in response to federal legislation, including the Best Pharmaceuticals for Children Act and the Pediatric Research Equity Act. Also, the National Institute for Mental Health began funding large, multisite treatment studies in the mid-1990s.

Currently, a number of medications are available with indications for psychiatric disorders in children, including ADHD, depression, obsessive-compulsive disorder, mania in bipolar disorder, psychosis in schizophrenia, and "irritability" in children with autism spectrum disorder. When prescribing these medications for other indications, and especially when prescribing a medication that has no indication for any psychiatric disorder in children and adolescents, the pediatric PCC should carefully justify and document the rationale in the medical record.

# FDA Boxed Warnings

Among stimulants and selective serotonin reuptake inhibitor (SSRIs), the most commonly prescribed psychotropic medications for youth, there is 1 boxed warning for SSRIs and 2 for stimulants. It is important to keep in mind that all adverse effects described in boxed warnings listed here occur infrequently and may never be seen by an individual pediatric PCC.

## SSRIs and Suicidality

The FDA boxed warning about suicidality for all antidepressants is a perceived obstacle for many pediatric PCCs who consider prescribing SSRIs for anxiety, depression, or both. The boxed warning stating that all antidepressants pose significant risk of suicidality (suicidal ideation or suicide attempts, not completed suicides) in children and adolescents was issued in October 2004. The warning recommended close monitoring for increased suicidality. Specific recommendations for monitoring were described in a medication guide provided by the FDA. The medication guide is a descriptive handout provided by pharmacists to inform parents or patients of indications, proper administration, and potential adverse effects of or concerns about a prescribed medication.

The medication guide included specific guidelines for monitoring, as follows: "your child should generally see his or her healthcare provider" weekly for the first 4 weeks, every 2 weeks for the next 4 weeks, at 12 weeks, and at the "healthcare provider's advice" after 12 weeks. This prescriptive monitoring mandate presented a major barrier to use of SSRIs in the primary care setting because this level of intensive monitoring is not compatible with most primary care practices.

In May 2007, the FDA issued a revised medication guide that no longer includes specific mandates for monitoring (www.fda.gov/downloads/Drugs /DrugSafety/InformationbyDrugClass/ucm100211.pdf). Instead, it focuses on information parents need to know regarding suicidality and antidepressants. Thus, the boxed warning should be regarded as just a warning, not a restriction.

Antidepressant-induced suicidality is rare. The original FDA estimate, based solely on data from more than 4,300 research participants in 23 studies, was that 2% of children and adolescents receiving placebo and 4% receiving an antidepressant developed suicidal thoughts or attempted suicide.[23] Thus, the risk difference was 2%. A subsequent analysis, based on data from 27 randomized controlled trials involving more than 5,300 participants, found a significant risk difference of just 0.7%.[24] The most recent estimate, which was based on data from 35 randomized controlled trials involving more than 6,000 participants, found a risk difference of 0.9%, just missing statistical significance.[25]

The most recent, and presumably best, analyses suggest that there may be a very slight increased risk of suicidality with antidepressants in children and adolescents. Clinical prudence indicates the need to educate patients and parents about suicidality and to provide careful monitoring for suicidality and other adverse effects during the initial phase of treatment (when risk of suicidality is generally greatest from both depression and medication) and throughout treatment.

## Stimulants and Cardiac Concerns

The boxed warning for amphetamine-based products states, "Misuse of amphetamines may cause sudden death and serious cardiovascular adverse effects." Methylphenidate-based products have a similar warning, but it is not "boxed." It is important to take a personal and family cardiac history, with emphasis on structural heart defects, syncope, sudden unexplained death, and arrhythmias, particularly long QT syndromes, before prescribing a stimulant for the first time. This screening is similar to that for sports physicals. A recent policy statement from the AAP[26] provides specific recommendations, including a "targeted cardiac history" and a "physical examination, including careful cardiac examination," "without obtaining routine electrocardiograms or routine subspecialty cardiology evaluations for most children."

## Stimulants and Concerns About Abuse and Dependence

The boxed warnings for amphetamines and methylphenidate state that they have a high potential for abuse and that prolonged administration may lead to dependence. Fortunately, there are no reports of children who were treated with therapeutic doses of stimulants developing dependence. Available data suggest that children with ADHD who are treated with stimulants are not more likely than those who did not receive stimulants to develop substance abuse later in life.[25,27,28] A related problem is diversion—that is, patients selling their prescription stimulants to be used as drugs of abuse.[29,30]

# References

1. A 14-month randomized clinical trial of treatment strategies for attention-deficit/ hyperactivity disorder. Multimodal Treatment Study of Children with ADHD. *Arch Gen Psychiatry.* 1999;56(12):1073–1086

2. Walkup JT, Albano AM, Piacentini J, et al. Cognitive behavioral therapy, sertraline, or a combination in childhood anxiety. *N Engl J Med.* 2008;359(26):2753–2766

3. March J, Silva S, Petrycki S, et al; Treatment for Adolescents With Depression Study (TADS) Team. Fluoxetine, cognitive-behavioral therapy, and their combination for adolescents with depression: Treatment for Adolescents with Depression Study (TADS) randomized controlled trial. *JAMA.* 2004;292(7):807–820

4. Gleason M, Egger L, Zeanah C, et al. Psychopharmacological treatment for very young children: contexts and guidelines. *J Am Acad Child Adolesc Psychiatry.* 2007;46(12): 1532–1572

5. Turner KM, Nicholson JM, Sanders MR. The role of practitioner self-efficacy, training, program and workplace factors on the implementation of an evidence-based parenting intervention in primary care. *J Primary Prevent.* 2011;32(2):95–112

6. McCormick E, Kerns SE, McPhillips H, Wright J, Christakis DA, Rivara FP. Training pediatric residents to provide parent education: a randomized control trial. *Academic Pediatrics.* 2014;14(4):353–360

7. Sanders MR, Ralph A, Sofronoff K, et al. Every family: a population approach to reducing behavioral and emotional problems in children making the transition to school. *J Primary Prevent.* 2008;29(3):197–222

8. Adam H, Foy J. *Signs and Symptoms in Pediatrics.* Elk Grove Village, IL: American Academy of Pediatrics; 2015

9. Stein RE, Horwitz SM, Storfer-Isser A, Heneghan A, Olson L, Hoagwood KE. Do pediatricians think they are responsible for identification and management of child mental health problems? Results of the AAP periodic survey. *Ambul Pediatr.* 2008;8(1):11–17

10. Kinderman KL. *Medicolegal Forms With Legal Analysis: Documenting Issues in the Patient-Physician Relationship.* 2nd ed. Chicago, IL: American Medical Association Press; 1999

11. American Academy of Child and Adolescent Psychiatry. Practice parameters on the use of psychotropic medication in children and adolescents. *J Am Acad Child Adoelsc Psychiatry.* 2009;48(9):961–973

12. World Health Organization. *Adherence to Long-term Therapies: Evidence for Action.* Geneva, Switzerland: World Health Organization; 2003

13. Case BG. Nonadherence: the silent majority. *J Am Acad Child Adoelsc Psychiatry.* 2011; 50(5):435–437

14. Pappadopulos E, Jensen PS, Chait AR, et al. Medication adherence in the MTA: saliva methylphenidate samples versus parent report and mediating effect of concomitant behavioral treatment. *J Am Acad Child Adolesc Psychiatry.* 2009;48(5):501–510

15. Olfson M, Marcus S, Wan G. Stimulant dosing for children with ADHD: a medical claims analysis. *J Am Acad Child Adoelsc Psychiatry.* 2009;48(1):51–59

16. Winterstein ADG, Gerhard T, Shuster J, Zito J, Johnson M, Liu H, Saidi A. Utilization of pharmacologic treatment in youths with attention deficit/hyperactivity disorder in Medicaid database. *Ann Pharmacother.* 2008;42(1):24–31

17. Charach A, Fernandez R. Enhancing ADHD medication adherence: challenges and opportunities. *Curr Psychiatry Rep.* 2013;15(7):371

18. Chong WW, Aslani P, Chen TF. Effectiveness of interventions to improve antidepressant medication adherence: a systematic review. *Int J Clin Pract.* 2011;65(9):954–975

19. Hamrin V, McGuinness TM. Motivational interviewing: a tool for increasing psychotropic medication adherence for youth. *J Psychosoc Nurs Ment Health Serv.* 2013;51(6): 15–18

20. McGuinness TM, Worley J. Promoting adherence to psychotropic medication for youth-part 1. *J Psychosoc Nurs Ment Health Serv.* 2010;48(10):19–22

21. McGuinness TM, Worley J. Promoting adherence to psychotropic medication for youth-part 2. *J Psychosoc Nurs Ment Health Serv.* 2010;48(10):22–26

22. Van Cleave J, Leslie LK. Approaching ADHD as a chronic condition: implications for long-term adherence. *J Psychosoc Nurs Ment Health Serv.* 2008;46(8):28–37

23. Bridge JA, Iyengar S, Salary CB, et al. Clinical response and risk for reported suicidal ideation and suicide attempts in pediatric antidepressant treatment: a meta-analysis of randomized controlled trials. *JAMA.* 2007;297(15):1683–1696

24. Hammad TA, Laughren T, Raccoosin J. Suicidality in pediatric patients treated with antidepressant drugs. *Arch Gen Psychiatry.* 2006;63(3):332–339

25. Mannuzza S, Klein RG, Troung NL, et al. Age of methylphenidate treatment initiation with ADHD and later substance abuse: prospective follow-up into adulthood. *Am J Psychiatry.* 2008;165(5):604–609

26. Perrin JM, Friedman RA, Knilans TK; American Academy of Pediatrics Black Box Working Group, Section on Cardiology and Cardiac Surgery. Cardiovascular monitoring and stimulant drugs for attentiondeficit/hyperactivity disorder. *Pediatrics.* 2008; 122(2):451–453

27. Wilson JJ. ADHD and substance use disorders: developmental aspects and the impact of stimulant treatment. *Am J Addict.* 2007;16(Suppl 1):5–11

28. Biederman J, Monuteaux MC, Spencer T, Wilens TE, Macpherson HA, Faraone SV. Stimulant therapy and risk for subsequent substance use disorders in male adults with ADHD: a naturalistic controlled 10-year follow-up study. *Am J Psychiatry.* 2008;165(5):597–603

29. Wilens TE, Adler LA, Adams J, et al. Misuse and diversion of stimulants prescribed for ADHD: a systematic review of the literature. *J Am Acad Child Adolesc Psychiatry.* 2008;47(1):21–31

30. Biederman J, Monuteaux MC, Spencer T, et al. Stimulant therapy and risk for subsequent substance use disorders in male adults with ADHD: a naturalistic controlled 10-year follow-up study. *Am J Psychiatry.* 2008;165:597–603

# Part 3—Group 1 Medications for Specific Diagnoses: ADHD, Anxiety, and Depression

# Group 1 Medications for Attention-Deficit/ Hyperactivity Disorder

## General Guidance

### Medications

Group 1 medications for attention-deficit/hyperactivity disorder (ADHD) belong to 3 classes. The rationale for using specific medications is similar to the overview in Chapter 1.

### *Stimulants*

Despite numerous products available on the market, just 2 are distinct stimulant chemical entities: *methylphenidate* and *amphetamine*. Both, in various preparations, are approved for treatment of ADHD in children and adolescents. The available literature has not shown advantages of different racemic mixtures (D- vs DL-). Thus, different racemic preparations are considered interchangeable, except for dose. Methylphenidate and amphetamine are available in numerous release preparations that provide a treatment effect ranging from 3 to 12 hours. Products with longer time on the market and lower cost may be preferred.

### $\alpha_2$-Adrenergic Agonists

*Guanfacine* is US Food and Drug Administration (FDA) approved for treatment of ADHD in children and adolescents. It is relatively specific to the $\alpha_{2A}$-receptor subtype, which is involved in attention regulation and impulse control. *Clonidine* is FDA approved for ADHD in children and adolescents. It nonspecifically interacts with $\alpha_{2A}$-, $\alpha_{2B}$-, and $\alpha_{2C}$-receptor subtypes. B and C receptors mediate sedation and hypotension and bradycardia adverse effects. Thus, clonidine may have a less favorable adverse effect profile than guanfacine; however, there are no direct comparative data regarding this issue. In addition, immediate-release (IR) (not sustained-release) clonidine is associated with acute drops in blood pressure, syncope, and even death following unintentional or intentional ingestions of more than therapeutic quantities.

## Norepinephrine Reuptake Inhibitor

*Atomoxetine*, a norepinephrine reuptake inhibitor, is also FDA approved for ADHD treatment. It has more concerning FDA warnings and precautions than other medications for ADHD included in Group 1.

## Reminder About Psychotherapies and Pragmatic Supports

Evidence-based and effective psychotherapies for youth with ADHD include behavioral management training for parents or caregivers and school personnel and social skills training for patients with problems in social interactions. In addition, consultation with school personnel is recommended.

In the United States, medication for ADHD is relatively common, while behavioral treatment is not. Recent data from the Centers of Disease Control and Prevention, focused on youth with special health needs,[1] indicate that 74% of youth with ADHD received medication *in the past week*, while only 44% received behavioral treatment *in the past year*. Only 31% received both past-week medication and past-year behavioral treatment.

## Choosing a Medication

Clinical guidance from the American Academy of Pediatrics (AAP)[2] and practice parameters from the American Academy of Child and Adolescent Psychiatry[3] recommend initiating medication with either of the stimulants, methylphenidate or amphetamine. Effect size (ie, magnitude of improvement relative to placebo) is greater for stimulants than other medications approved for ADHD. If there are concerns about starting with a stimulant (eg, specific potential adverse effents or parental preferences), guanfacine, clonidine, or atomoxetine are all secondary options with generally comparable therapeutic effect sizes.

*For preschool-aged children*, methylphenidate is recommended as the first medication for ADHD. There is only one National Institutes of Health–randomized, placebo-controlled study of any psychotropic medication for treatment of ADHD in preschool-aged children, the Preschool ADHD Treatment Study (PATS).[4] The PATS results indicate that, following a 10-week course of parent management training, IR methylphenidate, given 3 times a day in relatively low doses (optimal total daily dose ranged from

7.5 to 30 mg/day), was safe and effective in reducing symptoms of ADHD in preschoolers, aged 3 to 5 years. A 10- to 20-week trial of parental management training, parent-child interaction therapy, or both is recommended before considering methylphenidate for preschoolers with ADHD.[5] An amphetamine preparation is recommended if methylphenidate is ineffective or needs to be discontinued because of adverse effects. A follow-up of PATS participants found that most continued to receive medications for ADHD, primarily stimulants, over a 6-year follow-up period.[6]

## Adverse Effects: Boxed Warnings, Warnings and Precautions, and Adverse Reactions

Adverse effects can be evaluated based on either severity or frequency. Food and Drug Administration–required package inserts emphasize severity; thus, effects described as Boxed Warnings are more severe than Warnings and Precautions, which are more severe than Adverse Reactions. In addition, package inserts include Contraindications and Drug Interactions.

The most comprehensive and potentially least biased prescribing information about adverse effects can be found in FDA-required package inserts. They are available in various formats and locations, including

- Medication packaging
- *The Physician's Desk Reference*
- Online at Drugs@FDA

Since the FDA modified the format a few years ago, each label, or package insert, has a one-page *Highlights of Prescribing Information* that includes essential information about boxed warnings, warnings and precautions, adverse reactions, contraindications, and drug interactions. These highlights can be accessed and reviewed quickly and conveniently and are recommended as useful resources.

## Cost and Affordability

Historically, generic medications for ADHD, particularly stimulants, have been inexpensive. Recently, this has changed, and ADHD medications are a significant factor influencing cost of care for many pediatric populations. In an effort to control medication costs, many Medicaid programs and some private health plans provide formularies from which prescribing clinicians must select medications. Each plan's cost per prescription for the medications on these formularies depends on its contracts with the pharmaceutical suppliers. Generic medications may be in the same price range as—or even more expensive than—branded medications for which the plan has negotiated a favorable contract.

For uninsured and under-insured children, and for children whose families must make a co-payment at the time prescriptions are filled, the family's cost is a critical determinant of adherence. Responsibility falls to the prescriber to determine whether the family will experience financial barriers to filling prescriptions. Prescribers should inquire about the family's ability to purchase prescribed medications and should maintain an inventory of community resources for families unable to make co-pays or to purchase prescription medications. The pediatric primary care clinicians' (pediatric PCCs') staff can gather information about eligibility criteria and contact information for these resources. In some states, it may be necessary to refer the child into the behavioral health specialty system for the child to qualify.

## Information for Caregivers About Specific Medications

There are numerous sources of information about medications for patients, parents, and caregivers(s), as well other professionals, such as teachers and school nurses, who may have questions about medications. Many Web-based sources are supported, at least in part, by the pharmaceutical industry. The FDA *Patient Counseling Information* or *Medication Guide* is a useful and potentially less biased document located at the end of each package insert (available online at Drugs@FDA). This document should be given to the family by the pharmacist for all dispensed prescriptions, including those filled via mail order. In addition, the prescribing clinician can print the document and review it with the caregiver or patient.

# Methylphenidate Preparations

## Available Methylphenidate Preparations

Table 4.1 contains detailed information for the 13 methylphenidate preparations available on the US market, including

- Type of preparation
- Estimated duration of action
- Trade name
- Recommended initial dose
- Recommended maximum dose
- Available forms of the medication

Table 4.1. Methylphenidate Preparations

| Formulation | Duration[a] of effect, hours | Trade Name | Initial Dose | Max DD | Available Unit Dose Forms |
|---|---|---|---|---|---|
| Immediate-release (tablet) | 3–5 | Ritalin<br>Focalin | 5 and 5[b]<br>2.5 and 2.5[b] | 60<br>20 | 5, 10, or 20 mg<br>2.5, 5, or 10 mg |
| Pulse[c] (capsule) | 7–8 | Ritalin SR<br>Metadate ER<br>Methylin ER | 10[d]<br>10<br>10[d] | 60[d]<br>60<br>60[d] | 20 mg<br>10 or 20 mg<br>10 or 20 mg |
| Pearls (capsule) | 8–12 | Metadate CD<br>Ritalin LA<br>Focalin XR[e] | 20 (10[d])<br>20 (10[d])<br>5 | 60<br>60<br>30 | 10, 20, 30, 40, 50, or 60 mg<br>10, 20, 30, 40, or 60 mg<br>5, 10, 15, 20, 25, 30, 35, or 40 mg |
| Pump (capsule) | ≤12 | Concerta | 18 | 54 | 18, 27, 36, or 54 mg |
| Non-tablet or Non-capsule Formulations | | | | | |
| Chewable | 3–5 | Methylin | 5 and 5[b] | 60 | 2.5, 5, or 10 mg |
| Liquid | 3–5 | Methylin | 5 and 5[b] | 60 | 5 mg or 5 mL and 10 mg or 5 mL |
| Liquid | 8–12 | Quillivant XR[f] | 20 (10[d]) | 60 | 25 mg or 5 mL (in reconstituted form) |
| Transdermal patch | ≤12 | Daytrana[f] | 10 | (60[d]) | 10, 15, 20, or 30 mg (Each has about a 9-hour effect.) |

Abbreviation: max DD, maximum daily dose.

[a] Durations listed are based on the author's interpretation of available data, as well as the package insert.

[b] Immediate-release methylphenidate preparations are generally dosed at least twice a day, before breakfast and lunch.

[c] Pulse preparations are capsules containing a mixture of immediate-release beads and delayed-release beads. For children who cannot swallow capsules, they can be opened and the beads can be sprinkled into food such as applesauce.

[d] Author's recommendation, when information is not available in the package insert.

[e] Focalin is a dexmethylphenidate preparation; all others are racemic mixtures. Thus, dosing of Focalin is generally about one-half that of other methylphenidate preparations.

[f] Trade brand only (no generic available).

Classified using US Food and Drug Administration. Drugs@FDA Web site. http://www.accessdata.fda.gov/scripts/cder/drugsatfda. Accessed April 10, 2015.

Information in the table relies on FDA-approved package inserts or, when specific information is not available, on the author's recommendation.

The table is formatted to be relatively easy to use when seeking to gather comprehensive information about a specific medication: one can scan across the relevant row to find duration, initial dose, maximum dose, and available forms.

Because all methylphenidate preparations are controlled substances in the United States, a written (or approved electronic) prescription must be used for a maximum of a 30-day supply with no refills.

## Onset of Effect

Onset of effect for all methylphenidate preparations is generally 30 to 45 minutes. Appetite suppression occurs concurrently with therapeutic effect. Thus, timing of morning medication and breakfast needs to be coordinated.

## Duration of Effect

Four types of oral tablets and capsules are available. On average, IR preparations have a 3- to 5-hour duration of effect. The other 3 types have longer durations of effect, depending on technology used in the preparation: pulse or bead (7–8 hours), pearls (8–12 hours), or pump (≤12 hours). Duration of effect varies from child to child, and most estimates are based on aggregate group data. Familiarity with at least one preparation representing each type is recommended.

An obvious advantage of longer-acting preparations is once-daily dosing. This removes the stigmatizing effect of taking medication at school and improves adherence. Particularly if medication needs to be given very early (eg, 6:00 am or before the bus arrives), duration of effect of 7 to 8 hours may not be adequate for treating symptoms at school; a bus ride home or after-school child care may pose additional challenges for controlling symptoms. Duration of effect approximating 12 hours may be preferred in these instances and for children whose symptoms are a problem at home after the school day. Two potential problems with longer duration of effect are suppression of appetite and interference with sleep onset.

## Initial Dose

Table 4.1 presents recommended initial dose for all methylphenidate preparations. In general, the initial dose is 10 mg/day, once in the morning for long-acting preparations and two 5 mg doses of IR preparation separated by about 4 hours. Exceptions are dexmethylphenidate (Focalin) preparations, which require one-half the dose (ie, 5 mg once in the morning for the long-acting preparation or 2.5 mg twice a day for the IR preparation).

Lower initial dose is recommended for children younger than 6 years, ranging from about one-quarter to one-half of the initial doses in Table 4.1.

## Dosage Adjustments

Generally, dose can be increased weekly by an amount equivalent to the starting dose. An advantage of weekly adjustments is that parent and teacher ratings can be collected across school days and weekend days between dose adjustments. If there is a clear and positive response to the medication and no or minimal adverse effects, dose adjustments may be more frequent, as long as more frequent communication occurs with the caregiver(s) and school personnel.

## Monitoring Therapeutic Response During Dose Adjustments

During dose adjustment, a weekly phone check-in or appointment is preferred. Parent and teacher NICHQ Vanderbilt Assessment Scale reports can facilitate tracking change in severity of symptoms.

## Safety Monitoring

Monitoring for contraindications, adverse effects, and potential drug interactions starts before medication is prescribed and continues throughout drug administration. As with all medications, safety monitoring for methylphenidate depends on a targeted history and physical examination.

*Contraindications* include

- Known hypersensitivity to methylphenidate
- Marked anxiety, tension, or agitation
- Glaucoma
- Tics or a family history or diagnosis of Tourette syndrome (This contraindication is controversial.)
- Currently using, or within 2 weeks of using, a monoamine oxidase inhibitor (MAOI)

*Boxed warnings* include

- Concerns about abuse and dependence. A boxed warning for methylphenidate preparations states that it has a high potential for abuse and that prolonged administration may lead to dependence. Fortunately, there are no reports of children who were treated with therapeutic doses of stimulants developing dependence. Available data suggest that children with ADHD who are treated with stimulants are not more likely than those who did not receive stimulants to develop substance abuse later in life.[7-9] A related problem is diversion—that is, patients selling their prescription stimulants to be used as drugs of abuse.[10]

*Warnings and precautions:* Most warnings and precautions rarely occur in children and adolescents treated with stimulants. Those most relevant to youth taking methylphenidate preparations include

- Increase in blood pressure and heart rate (most common)
- Serious cardiovascular events (generally only in patients with known structural cardiac abnormalities, cardiomyopathy, serious heart rhythm abnormalities, coronary artery disease, or other serious heart problems) (A detailed personal and family cardiac history is important, with emphasis on the presence of structural heart defects, syncope, sudden unexplained death, and arrhythmias, particularly long QT syndromes, before prescribing any ADHD medication, including stimulants. A recent policy statement from the AAP[11] provides specific recommendations, including a "targeted cardiac history" plus a "physical examination, including careful cardiac examination," "without obtaining routine ECGs [electrocardiograms] or routine subspecialty cardiology evaluations" for most children.)
- Psychiatric events (primarily emergence of psychotic, manic, or aggressive symptoms [or a combination of those])
- Seizures
- Long-term growth suppression
- Exacerbation of tics
- Priapism

*Adverse reactions:* Across the package inserts for various methylphenidate preparations is variation in the adverse effects listed. Those reported most consistently are

- Abdominal pain
- Appetite suppression
- Insomnia

*Drug interactions* may occur with MAOIs (current or within past 2 weeks; various symptoms), vasopressors (increased blood pressure), or coumadin anticoagulants, as well as some anticonvulsants (methylphenidate inhibits their metabolism).

## Vital Signs, Physical Examination, and Laboratory Monitoring

For all stimulants, monitoring blood pressure, heart rate, height, and weight is recommended. In addition, patients taking stimulants should be observed for, and parents should be questioned about, tics. No specific laboratory studies are recommended.

## Optimizing Dose

A general recommendation for optimizing dose—if confident that the child has adhered to the previously prescribed dose—is to continue to increase the dose until the benefit-to-risk ratio is optimized. Treatment response, assessed systematically using information from parent and teacher reports (eg, NICHQ Vanderbilt Assessment Scale ratings), should be considered alongside reported and observed adverse effects during dose escalation. Satisfaction of the caregiver, teacher, and child regarding the child's response can also be useful. Ideally, a consensus will emerge about the preferred dose that maximizes the benefit-to-risk ratio.

## Maintenance

Once an optimal dose is determined, maintenance treatment begins. Frequency of monitoring can be reduced, usually to follow-ups every 1 to 3 months, depending on the patient's needs. Consideration of dose adjustments is recommended annually or more often if the patient's clinical status changes significantly.

## Medication Holidays

Particularly for patients with methylphenidate-induced growth suppression, medication "holidays" may be beneficial. Discontinuation of medication during a summer school recess may be sufficient to allow a growth "rebound."

## What if a Methylphenidate Preparation Is Ineffective or Not Tolerated?

If adverse effects limit sufficient dose escalation or if the initial medication is not considered sufficiently beneficial, discontinuation is recommended.

If continued medication treatment is clinically indicated, consideration of another ADHD medication may be warranted. Available data suggest that a methylphenidate or an amphetamine preparation is effective in almost all children, so switching from one to the other is generally indicated if the first is ineffective.

## Discontinuing Methylphenidate and Possible Withdrawal Adverse Effects

For most patients, particularly those receiving extended-release (ER) preparations at recommended dosages, methylphenidate can be discontinued abruptly. To minimize withdrawal adverse effects, particularly for patients receiving high doses, staggered discontinuation of methylphenidate over a few days to weeks is recommended. Potential withdrawal adverse effects include anxiety, irritability, insomnia, and increased blood pressure.

## Switching From a Methylphenidate to an Amphetamine Preparation

Switching from a methylphenidate preparation to a comparable amphetamine one can be done abruptly or over a few days, as long as the total daily dose is clinically comparable (ie, the amphetamine dose is about one-half the methylphenidate one).

## When to Consult or Refer

In general, consultation with, or referral to, a child and adolescent psychiatrist or other prescribing specialist may be considered when there is lack of clarity about diagnosis or after several medications have been tried and discontinued because of lack of effect or tolerability. A more extensive discussion regarding what to do when interventions fail is presented in Chapter 8.

# Amphetamine Preparations

## Available Amphetamine Preparations

Amphetamine preparations available in the United States are listed in Table 4.2 along with

- Type of preparation
- Estimated duration of action
- Trade name

- Recommended initial dose
- Recommended maximum dose
- Available dosage forms of the medication

Information in the table relies on FDA-approved labels (package inserts) or, when specific information is not available, on the author's recommendation.

*Vyvanse* deserves additional consideration because of several characteristics. The amount of D-amphetamine in each Vyvanse capsule is not available in the package insert. Thus, it is difficult to convert to comparable doses of other stimulants. In addition, onset of the effects of Vyvanse may be delayed by about 30 to 60 minutes compared with other stimulants because absorption of the lysine-dextroamphetamine molecule is taken up more slowly than regular D-amphetamine, which is rapidly absorbed via an active transporter in the gastrointestinal tract. Almost immediately after reaching the blood stream, the lysine-dextroamphetamine bond is cleaved, releasing regular D-amphetamine. Claims regarding lack of abuse potential for Vyvanse compared with other amphetamine preparations are technically correct because it is ineffective if taken intravenously or by nasal snorting; this may be an important consideration in instances when there is a risk of diversion of the prescribed medication to substance abusers but may not be important to most pediatric patients.

Because all methylphenidate preparations are controlled substances in the United States, a written (or approved electronic) prescription must be used for a maximum of a 30-day supply with no refills.

## Onset of Effect

Onset of effect for all amphetamine preparations (except possibly Vyvanse) is generally 30 to 45 minutes. In addition to therapeutic effects, appetite suppression occurs concurrently. Thus, timing of morning medication and breakfast needs to be coordinated.

## Duration of Effect

Four types of oral tablets and capsules are available. On average, IR preparations have a 4- to 8-hour duration of effect. The other 3 types have longer durations of effect, depending on technology used in the preparation: pulse or bead (7–8 hours), pearls (8–12 hours), or prodrug (≤12 hours). Duration of effect varies from child to child; most estimates are based on aggregate

**Table 4.2. D-Amphetamine and DL-Amphetamine (Mixed-Salt) Preparations**

| Formulation | Form | Duration[a] of effect (hours) | Trade Name | Initial Dose | Max DD | Available Unit Dose Forms |
|---|---|---|---|---|---|---|
| Immediate Release[b] | D-tablet | 4–8 | Zenzedi | 5 and 5[b] | 40 | 2.5 5 7.5 10 15 20 30 |
| Immediate Release[b] | DL-tablet | 4–8 | Adderall Evekeo | 5 and 5[b] | 40 | 5, 7.5, 10, 12.5, 15, 20, or 30 mg 5 and 10 mg |
| Pulse[c] | D-capsule | 6–9 | Dexedrine Spansule | 5 | 40 | 5, 10, or 15 mg |
| Pearl | DL-capsule | 8–12 | Adderall XR | 10 (5[d]) | 30 | 5, 10, 15, 20, 25, or 30 mg |
| Modified IR ("prodrug") | D-capsule | 8–12 | Vyvanse[e] | 20 | 70 | 20, 30, 40, 50, 60, or 70 mg |
| **Non-tablet or Non-capsule Formulations** | | | | | | |
| IR[b] | D-liquid | ≤8 | ProCentra[e] | 5 | 40 | 5 mL or 5 cc |

Abbreviation: IR, immediate-release; max DD, maximum daily dose.

[a] Durations listed are based on the author's interpretation of available data, as well as the package insert.

[b] Recommended starting dose is twice daily, about 4–6 hours apart.

[c] Pulse preparations are capsules containing a mixture of immediate-release beads and delayed-release beads. For children who cannot swallow capsules, they can be opened and the beads can be sprinkled into food such as applesauce.

[d] Author's recommendation.

[e] Trade brand only (no generic available).

Classified using US Food and Drug Administration. Drugs@FDA Web site. http://www.accessdata.fda.gov/scripts/cder/drugsatfda. Accessed April 10, 2015.

group data. Familiarity with at least one preparation representing each type is recommended.

An obvious advantage of longer-acting preparations is once-daily dosing; this removes the stigmatizing effect of taking medication at school and improves adherence. Particularly if medication needs to be given very early (eg, 6:00 am or before the bus arrives), duration of effect of less than about 8 hours may not be adequate for treating symptoms at school; a bus ride home or after-school child care may pose additional challenges for controlling symptoms. Duration of effect approximating 12 hours may be preferred in these instances and for children whose symptoms are a problem at home after the school day.

## Initial Dose

Table 4.2 presents recommended initial dose for all amphetamine preparations. In general, dosing of amphetamine preparations is about one-half that of methylphenidate. In general, the initial dose is 5 to 10 mg/day, once in the morning for long-acting preparations and two 2.5-mg or 5-mg doses separated by about 4 to 6 hours for IR.

Lower initial dose is recommended for children younger than 6 years, ranging from about one-quarter to one-half the initial doses in Table 4.2.

## Dosage Adjustments

Generally, dose can be increased weekly by an amount equivalent to the starting dose. An advantage of weekly adjustments is that parent and teacher ratings can be collected across school days and weekend days between dose adjustments. If there is a clear and positive response to the medication and no or minimal adverse effects, dose adjustments may be more frequent, as long as more frequent communication occurs with the caregiver(s) and school personnel.

## Monitoring Therapeutic Response During Dose Adjustments

During dose adjustment, a weekly phone check-in or appointment is preferred. Parent and teacher NICHQ Vanderbilt Assessment Scale reports can facilitate tracking change in severity of symptoms.

## Safety Monitoring

Monitoring for contraindications, adverse effects, and potential drug interactions starts before medication is prescribed and continues throughout drug administration. As with all medications, safety monitoring for amphetamine depends on a targeted history and physical examination.

*Contraindications* include

- Advanced atherosclerosis
- Symptomatic cardiovascular disease
- Moderate-to-severe hypertension
- Hyperthyroidism
- Known hypersensitivity or idiosyncratic reaction to the sympathomimetic amines
- Glaucoma
- Agitated states
- History of drug abuse
- Currently using, or within 2 weeks of using, an MAOI

*Boxed warnings* include

- Cardiac concerns. The boxed warning for amphetamine-based products states: "Misuse of amphetamines may cause sudden death and serious cardiovascular adverse effects." A detailed personal and family cardiac history is important, with emphasis on presence of structural heart defects, syncope, sudden unexplained death, and arrhythmias, particularly long QT syndromes, before prescribing any ADHD medication, including stimulants. A recent policy statement from the AAP[11] provides specific recommendations, including a "targeted cardiac history" plus a "physical examination, including careful cardiac examination," "without obtaining routine ECGs [electrocardiograms] or routine subspecialty cardiology evaluations" for most children.
- Concerns about abuse and dependence. The boxed warnings for amphetamines state that they have a high potential for abuse and that prolonged administration may lead to dependence. Fortunately, there are no reports of children who were treated with therapeutic doses of stimulants developing dependence. Available data suggest that children with ADHD who are treated with stimulants are not more likely than those who did not receive stimulants to develop substance abuse later in life.[7-9] A related problem is diversion—that is, patients selling their prescription stimulants to be used as drugs of abuse.[10]

*Warnings and precautions:* Most warnings and precautions rarely occur in children and adolescents treated with stimulants. Those most relevant to youth taking amphetamine preparations include

- Increase in blood pressure (most common)
- Serious cardiovascular events (generally only in patients with known structural cardiac abnormalities, cardiomyopathy, serious heart rhythm abnormalities, coronary artery disease, or other serious heart problems)
- Psychiatric events (primarily emergence of psychotic, manic, or aggressive symptoms [or a combination of those])
- Seizures
- Long-term growth suppression
- Exacerbation of tics

*Adverse reactions:* Across the package inserts for various amphetamine preparations, there is variation in the adverse effects listed. Those reported most consistently are

- Abdominal pain
- Appetite suppression
- Insomnia
- Weight loss
- Nervousness

*Drug interactions* include

- Monoamine oxidases (current or within 14 days) *may potentiate* the effects of amphetamine.
- Alkalinizing agents *may increase* blood levels of amphetamine.
- Acidifying agents *may reduce* blood levels of amphetamine.
- Effects of α-adrenergic blocking agents, antihistamines, antihypertensives, phenobarbital, phenytoin, Veratrum alkaloids, and ethosuximide *may be reduced* by amphetamine.
- Effects of tricyclic antidepressants, norepinephrine, and meperidine *may be potentiated* by amphetamine.

## Vital Signs, Physical Examination, and Laboratory Monitoring

For all amphetamine preparations, monitoring blood pressure, heart rate, height, and weight is recommended. In addition, patients taking stimulants should be observed for, and parents should be questioned about, tics. No specific laboratory studies are recommended.

## Optimizing Dose

A general recommendation for optimizing dose—if confident that the child has adhered to the previously prescribed dose—is to continue to increase the dose until the benefit-to-risk ratio is optimized. Treatment response, assessed systematically using information from parent and teacher reports (eg, NICHQ Vanderbilt Assessment Scale ratings), should be considered alongside reported and observed adverse effects during dose escalation. Satisfaction of the caregiver, teacher, and child regarding the child's response can also be useful. Ideally, a consensus will emerge about the preferred dose that maximizes the benefit-to-risk ratio.

## Maintenance

Once an optimal dose is determined, maintenance treatment begins. Frequency of monitoring can be reduced, usually to follow-ups every 1 to 3 months, depending on the patient's needs. Consideration of dose adjustments is recommended annually, or more often, if the patient's clinical status changes significantly.

## Medication Holidays

Particularly for patients with amphetamine-induced growth suppression, medication "holidays" may be beneficial. Discontinuation of medication during a summer school recess may be sufficient to allow a growth "rebound."

## What if an Amphetamine Preparation Is Ineffective or Not Tolerated?

If adverse effects limit sufficient dose escalation or if the initial medication is not considered sufficiently beneficial, discontinuation is recommended. If continued medication treatment is clinically indicated, consideration of another ADHD medication may be warranted. Available data suggest that a methylphenidate or an amphetamine preparation is effective in almost all children, so switching from one to the other is generally indicated if the first is ineffective.

## Discontinuing Amphetamine and Possible Withdrawal Adverse Effects

For most patients, particularly those receiving ER preparations at recommended dosages, amphetamine can be discontinued abruptly. To minimize withdrawal adverse effects, particularly for patients receiving high doses, staggered discontinuation of amphetamine over a few days to weeks is recommended. Potential withdrawal adverse effects include anxiety, irritability, insomnia, and increased blood pressure.

## Switching From an Amphetamine to a Methylphenidate Preparation
Switching from an amphetamine preparation to a comparable methylphenidate one can be done abruptly or over a few days, as long as the total daily dose is clinically comparable (ie, the methylphenidate dose is about twice the amphetamine one).

## When to Consult or Refer
In general, consultation with, or referral to, a child and adolescent psychiatrist or other prescribing specialist may be considered when there is lack of clarity about diagnosis or after several medications have been tried and discontinued because of lack of effect or tolerability. A more extensive discussion regarding what to do when interventions fail is presented in Chapter 8.

# Guanfacine Preparations

## Available Guanfacine Preparations
Guanfacine is an $\alpha_{2A}$-adrenergic agonist. Guanfacine preparations available in the United States are listed in Table 4.3 along with

- Type of preparation
- Estimated duration of action
- Trade name
- Recommended initial dose
- Recommended maximum dose
- Available forms of the medication

Information in the table relies on FDA-approved labels (package inserts) or, occasionally, the author's recommendation when specific information is not available.

Extended-release guanfacine (generic and Intuniv) is FDA approved for ADHD in children, adolescents, and adults, aged 6 and older. Immediate-release guanfacine (generic and Tenex) is approved for management of hypertension in adults. Because all guanfacine preparations have the same active agent and are used to treat ADHD in youth, they are included here.

**Table 4.3. Guanfacine Preparations**

| Drug | Formulation | Duration[a] of effect (hours) | Trade Name | Initial Dose | Max DD | Available Unit Dose Forms |
|------|-------------|-------------------------------|------------|--------------|--------|---------------------------|
| Guanfacine | IR | 4–8 | Tenex | 0.5-1.0[b] | 4 (divided)[b] | 1 or 2 mg tablets |
| Guanfacine | ER[c] | ≤24 | Intuniv | 1 | 7 | 1, 2, 3, or 4 mg tablets |

Abbreviations: ER, extended-release; IR, immediate-release; max DD, maximum daily dose.

[a] Durations listed are based on the author's interpretation of available data, as well as the package insert.

[b] Author's recommendation.

[c] For extended-release guanfacine, once-daily dosing is recommended.

Classified using US Food and Drug Administration. Drugs@FDA Web site. http://www.accessdata.fda.gov/scripts/cder/drugsatfda. Accessed April 10, 2015.

An advantage of the ER preparation is its "flatter" pharmacokinetic profile (ie, the peak level is relatively lower and thus may be associated with fewer or lesser adverse effects than comparable IR preparations).[12(figure1)] A disadvantage is that, at the present time, generic and brand ER guanfacine preparations are significantly more costly than IR guanfacine preparations.

Several points in the ER guanfacine package insert[12(p1)] regarding administration are noteworthy.

- "Do not crush, chew, or break tablets before swallowing."
- "Do not administer with high-fat meals, because of increased exposure."
- "Do not substitute for immediate-release guanfacine tablets on a mg-per-mg basis, because of differing pharmacokinetic profiles."

## Onset of Effect

Precise data regarding onset of effect of guanfacine preparations are not available. Clinical experience suggests therapeutic effects occur within 1 to 2 hours after administration.

## Duration of Effect

Immediate-release guanfacine has a 4- to 8-hour duration of effect. Duration of effect of ER guanfacine is up to 24 hours. The higher the dose, the longer the potential effects, both therapeutic and adverse. Duration of effect varies from child to child; the estimates in Table 4.3 are group ones.

An obvious advantage of longer-acting preparations is once-daily dosing; this removes the stigmatizing effect of taking medication at school and improves adherence. Particularly if medication needs to be given very early (eg, 6:00 am or before the bus arrives), duration of effect of 7 to 8 hours may not be adequate for treating symptoms at school; a bus ride home or after-school child care may pose additional challenges for controlling symptoms. Duration of effect approximating 12 hours may be preferred in these instances and for children whose symptoms are a problem at home after the school day. Two potential problems with longer duration of effect are sedation and somnolence.

## Initial Dose

The recommended starting dose of ER guanfacine is 1 mg, either in the morning or evening. Because IR guanfacine is approved only for hypertension in adults, no relevant dosing recommendations for youth with ADHD are in the package insert. Clinical experience and expert opinion suggest starting with 0.5 mg (one-half of 1-mg tablet) or 1 mg in the morning.

Guanfacine, in any formulation, is not FDA approved for use in youth younger than 6 years. In these patients, if stimulants are ineffective or not tolerated, consultation with a specialist regarding reconsideration of diagnosis and next steps in treatment is recommended.

The lowest dose available of ER guanfacine is 1 mg.

## Dosage Adjustments

Generally, dose can be increased weekly by an amount equivalent to the starting dose. An advantage of weekly adjustments is that parent and teacher ratings can be collected across school days and weekend days between dose adjustments. If there is a clear and positive response to the medication and no or minimal adverse effects, dose adjustments may be more frequent, as long as more frequent communication with the caregiver(s) and school personnel occurs.

In monotherapy clinical trials of ER guanfacine,

> There was dose- and exposure-related clinical improvement as well as risks for several clinically significant adverse effects (hypotension, bradycardia, sedative events). To balance the exposure-related potential benefits and risks, the recommended target dose range depending on clinical response and tolerability for Intuniv is 0.05–0.12 mg/kg/day (*total daily dose between 1–7 mg*). . . . In adjunctive trial which evaluated Intuniv treatment with psychostimulants, the majority of patients reached optimal doses in the 0.05–0.12 mg/kg/day range. Doses above 4 mg/day have not been studied in adjunctive trials.[12(p3)]

Because IR guanfacine is approved only for hypertension in adults, there are no relevant dosing recommendations for youth with ADHD in the package insert. Clinical experience and expert opinion suggest a maximum total daily dose of 4 mg, which is the recommended maximum for treatment of hypertension in adults.

## Monitoring Therapeutic Response During Dose Adjustments

During dose adjustment, a weekly phone check-in or appointment is preferred. Parent and teacher NICHQ Vanderbilt Assessment Scale reports can facilitate tracking change in severity of symptoms.

# Safety Monitoring

Monitoring for contraindications, adverse effects, and potential drug inter-actions starts before medication is prescribed and continues throughout drug administration. As with all medications, safety monitoring for guanfacine depends on a targeted history and physical examination. The information below is based on the package insert for Intuniv,[12] which is derived, in part, from clinical trials involving youth, aged 6 to 17.

*The only contraindication* is history of hypersensitivity to Intuniv or other guanfacine products.

*Boxed warnings:* There are no boxed warnings.

*Warnings and precautions*[12(p1)] are

> *Hypotension, bradycardia, syncope:* Titrate slowly and monitor vital signs fre-quently in patients at risk for hypotension, heart block, bradycardia, syncope, cardiovascular disease, vascular disease, cerebrovascular disease, or chronic renal failure. Measure heart rate and blood pressure prior to initiation of therapy, following dose increases, and periodically while on therapy. Avoid concomitant use of drugs with additive effects unless clinically indicated. Advise patients to avoid becoming dehydrated or overheated.

> *Sedation and somnolence:* Occur commonly with Intuniv. Consider the potential for additive effects with CNS [central nervous system] depressant drugs. Caution patients against operating heavy equipment or driving until they know how they respond to Intuniv. [Examples of central nervous system depressants: alcohol, barbiturates, benzodiazepines.]

> *Cardiac conduction abnormalities:* May worsen sinus node dysfunction and atrioventricular (AV) block, especially in patients taking other sympatholytic agents. Titrate slowly and monitor vital signs frequently.

*Adverse reactions:* Most common (>5% and at least twice the placebo rate) in Intuniv fixed-dose monotherapy ADHD trials in 6- to 17-year-olds are

- Hypotension
- Somnolence
- Fatigue
- Nausea
- Lethargy

Additional adverse effects in Intuniv flexible dose–optimization ADHD trials were abdominal pain, insomnia, dizziness, dry mouth, irritability, vomiting, and bradycardia.

*Drug interactions* include

- "Strong CYP3A4 inhibitors increase guanfacine exposure. [Examples of 'strong' (clarithromycin, ketoconazole, nefazodone) and 'moderate' (doxycycline, fluvoxamine, grapefruit juice) CYP3A4 inhibitors.]"
- "Strong CYP3A4 inducers decrease guanfacine exposure. [Examples of CYP3A4 inducers: barbiturates, carbamazepine, glucocorticoids, phenytoin, St. John's wort.]"

## Vital Signs and Laboratory Monitoring

For all guanfacine preparations, monitoring blood pressure and heart rate is recommended. No specific laboratory studies are recommended.

## Optimizing Dose

A general recommendation for optimizing dose—if confident that the child has adhered to the previously prescribed dose—is to continue to increase the dose until the benefit-to-risk ratio is optimized. Treatment response, assessed systematically using information from parent and teacher reports (eg, NICHQ Vanderbilt Assessment Scale ratings), should be considered alongside reported and observed adverse effects during dose escalation. Satisfaction of the caregiver, teacher, and child regarding the child's response can also be useful. Ideally, a consensus will emerge about the preferred dose that maximizes the benefit-to-risk ratio.

Specifics regarding optimizing dose were presented in the previous Dosage Adjustments section.

## Maintenance

Once an optimal dose is determined, maintenance treatment begins. Frequency of monitoring can be reduced, usually to follow-ups every 1 to 3 months, depending on the patient's needs. Consideration of dose adjustments is recommended annually, or more often, if the patient's clinical status changes significantly.

## What if a Guanfacine Preparation Is Ineffective or Not Tolerated?

If adverse effects limit sufficient dose escalation or if the maximal recommended dose is ineffective, discontinuation is recommended. If continued medication is clinically indicated, consideration of another class of ADHD medication may be warranted.

## Discontinuing Guanfacine and Possible Withdrawal Adverse Effects

To minimize withdrawal adverse effects, it is recommended that IR and ER guanfacine be tapered in daily dose increments of 1 mg every 3 to 7 days. Blood pressure and pulse monitoring is recommended during taper and discontinuation.

Potential withdrawal adverse effects include small increases in blood pressure and heart rate.

## Switching From One to Another Guanfacine Preparation

The following text is taken verbatim from the Intuniv package insert[12(p3)]:

> If switching from immediate-release guanfacine, discontinue that treatment, and titrate Intuniv following the above recommended schedule. [See summary in the previous Dosage Adjustments section.] . . . Do not substitute for immediate-release guanfacine tablets on a milligram-per-milligram basis, because of differing pharmacokinetic profiles. Intuniv has significantly reduced Cmax [maximum serum concentration] (60% lower), bioavailability (43% lower) and a delayed Tmax [time of maximum serum concentration] (3 hours later) compared to those of the same dose of immediate-release guanfacine.

Thus, in general, a 1-mg dose of IR guanfacine would be approximately equivalent to a 1.5-mg dose of ER guanfacine.

## Adjunct Treatment to Stimulants

Extended-release guanfacine is FDA approved for adjunctive treatment to stimulants. This may be considered when the stimulant dose cannot be optimized because of adverse effects in the context of persisting ADHD symptoms. Recommendations for using adjunctive guanfacine preparations are the same as when it is used alone. It is important to note that combination treatment may be prone to a higher likelihood of adverse effects and that, in general, treatment with one medication is preferable, when possible.

## When to Consult or Refer

In general, consultation with, or referral to, a child and adolescent psychiatrist or other prescribing specialist may be considered when there is lack of clarity about diagnosis or after several medications have been tried and discontinued because of lack of effect or tolerability. A more extensive discussion regarding what to do when interventions fail is presented in Chapter 8.

# Clonidine Preparations

## Available Clonidine Preparations

Clonidine is an $\alpha_2$-adrenergic agonist. Clonidine is available in the United States in 3 forms: IR tablets (Catapres and generic), ER tablets (Kapvay and generic [ER clonidine]), and transdermal patch (Catapres-TTS). Kapvay and ER clonidine are the only clonidine formulations approved for treatment of ADHD in youth 6 to 17 years. Catapres and generic formulations are approved for treatment of hypertension in adults. Because all clonidine preparations have the same active agent and are used to treat ADHD in youth, they are included here (Table 4.4).

ER clonidine is FDA approved for ADHD in children and adolescents. Clonidine nonspecifically interacts with $\alpha_{2A}$-, $\alpha_{2B}$-, and $\alpha_{2C}$-receptor subtypes. The 2B receptor mediates, via baroreceptors, hypotension and bradycardia adverse effects. Thus, clonidine may have a less favorable adverse effect profile than guanfacine. There are no direct comparative data regarding this issue. In addition, IR clonidine is associated with acute drops in blood pressure, syncope, and even death following unintentional or intentional ingestions of more than therapeutic quantities.

Clonidine preparations available in the United States are listed in Table 4.4 along with

- Type of preparation
- Estimated duration of action
- Trade name
- Recommended initial dose
- Recommended maximum dose
- Available forms of the medication

Information in the table relies on FDA-approved package inserts or, occasionally, the author's recommendation when specific information is not available.

**Table 4.4. Clonidine Preparations**

| Drug | Formulation | Duration[a] of effect (hours) | Trade Name | Initial Dose | Max DD | Available Unit Dose Forms |
|---|---|---|---|---|---|---|
| Clonidine | IR | 3–5 | Catapres | 0.05[b] | 0.4 (divided) | 0.1, 0.2, or 0.3 mg tablets |
| Clonidine | ER[c] | 12-24[b] | Kapvay | 0.1 hs | 0.4 (divided) | 0.1 or 0.2 mg tablets |
| **Non-tablet or Non-capsule Formulations** | | | | | | |
| Clonidine | Patch | 7 days | Catapres | 0.05[b] | 0.3[b] | 0.1, 0.2, or 0.3 mg/day |

Abbreviations: ER, extended-release; IR, immediate-release; Max DD, maximum daily dose.
[a] Durations listed are based on the author's interpretation of available data, as well as the package insert.
[b] Author's recommendation.
[c] For extended-release clonidine, twice-a-day dosing is recommended.
Classified using US Food and Drug Administration. Drugs@FDA Web site. http://www.accessdata.fda.gov/scripts/cder/drugsatfda. Accessed April 10, 2015.

An advantage of the ER preparation is its "flatter" pharmacokinetic profile, (ie, the peak level is relatively lower and thus may be associated with fewer or lesser adverse effects than comparable IR clonidine).[13(Figure1)] A disadvantage is that no generic ER clonidine is available.

Several points in the Kapvay package insert[13(P1)] regarding administration are noteworthy.

- "Do not crush, chew, or break tablets before swallowing."
- "Do not substitute for other clonidine products on a mg-per-kg basis, because of differing pharmacokinetic profiles."
- "When discontinuing, taper the dose in decrements of no more than 0.1 mg every 3 to 7 days to avoid rebound hypotension."

These points are discussed in the Dosage Adjustments section.

## Onset of Effect

Precise data regarding onset of effect of clonidine preparations is not available. Clinical experience suggests therapeutic effects occur generally within 30 to 60 minutes after administration.

## Duration of Effect

Immediate-release clonidine has a 3- to 5-hour duration of effect. The duration of effect of ER clonidine is 12 to 24 hours. The higher the dose, the longer the potential effects, both therapeutic and adverse. Duration of effect varies from child to child; the estimates in Table 4.3 are group estimates.

An obvious advantage of ER preparations is once-daily dosing (which is an option with ER clonidine, despite the suggested twice-a-day dosing in the package insert); this removes the stigmatizing effect of taking medication at school and improves adherence. Particularly if medication needs to be given very early (eg, 6:00 am or before the bus arrives), duration of effect of less than about 8 hours may not be adequate for treating symptoms at school; a bus ride home or after-school child care may pose additional challenges for controlling symptoms. Duration of effect approximating 12 hours may be preferred in these instances and for children whose symptoms are a problem at home after the school day.

## Initial Dose

The recommended starting dose of ER clonidine is 0.1 mg at bedtime. Because IR clonidine is approved only for hypertension in adults, there are no relevant dosing recommendations for youth with ADHD in the package insert. Clinical experience and expert opinion suggest starting with 0.05 mg in the morning or at bedtime.

Clonidine, in any formulation, is not FDA approved for use in youth younger than 6 years. In these patients, if stimulants are ineffective or not tolerated, consultation with a specialist regarding reconsideration of diagnosis and next steps in treatment is recommended.

## Dosage Adjustments

Generally, dose can be increased weekly by an amount equivalent to the starting dose. An advantage of weekly adjustments is that parent and teacher ratings can be collected across school days and weekend days between dose adjustments. If there is a clear and positive response to the medication and no or minimal adverse effects, dose adjustments may be more frequent, as long as more frequent communication occurs with the caregiver(s) and school personnel.

> The dose of Kapvay, administered either as monotherapy or as adjunctive therapy to a psychostimulant, should be individualized according to the therapeutic needs and response of the patient. Dosing should be initiated with one 0.1 mg tablet at bedtime, and the daily dosage should be adjusted in increments of 0.1 mg/day at weekly intervals until the desired response is achieved. Doses should be taken twice a day, with either an equal or higher split dosage being given at bedtime.[13(Section2.3,p3)]

The maximum recommended total daily dose is 0.4 mg. Because IR clonidine is approved only for hypertension in adults, there are no relevant dosing recommendations for youth with ADHD in the package insert. Clinical experience and expert opinion suggest a maximum total daily dose of 0.4 mg, which is the recommended maximum for treatment of hypertension in adults. Dosing may be up to 4 times a day, depending on patient need; no single dose should exceed 0.2 mg.

## Monitoring Therapeutic Response During Dose Adjustments

During dose adjustment, a weekly phone check-in or appointment is preferred. Parent and teacher NICHQ Vanderbilt Assessment Scale reports can facilitate tracking change in severity of symptoms.

## Safety Monitoring

Monitoring for contraindications, adverse effects, and potential drug inter-actions starts before medication is prescribed and continues throughout drug administration. As with all medications, safety monitoring for clonidine depends on a targeted history and physical examination. The information below is based on the package insert for Kapvay.[13] The safety data for this package insert is derived, in part, from clinical trials involving youth, aged 6 to 17.

*The only contraindication* is history of hypersensitivity reaction to clonidine.

*Boxed warnings:* There are no boxed warnings.

*Warnings and precautions* (verbatim from package insert)[13(p1)] are

> *Hypotension, bradycardia, syncope:* Titrate slowly and monitor vital signs frequently in patients at risk for hypotension, heart block, bradycardia, syncope, cardiovascular disease, vascular disease, cerebrovascular disease or chronic renal failure. Measure heart rate and blood pressure prior to initiation of therapy, following dose increases, and periodically while on therapy. Avoid concomitant use of drugs with additive effects unless clinically indicated. Advise patients to avoid becoming dehydrated or overheated.

> *Somnolence/sedation:* Has been observed with Kapvay. Consider the potential for additive effects with CNS [central nervous system] depressant drugs. Caution patients against operating heavy equipment or driving until they know how they respond to Kapvay.

> *Cardiac conduction abnormalities:* May worsen sinus node dysfunction and atrioventricular (AV) block, especially in patients taking other sympatholytic agents. Titrate slowly and monitor vital signs frequently.

*Adverse reactions:* Most common (>5% and at least twice the placebo rate) in monotherapy trials of ADHD in 6- to 17-year-olds are

- Somnolence
- Fatigue
- Irritability
- Nightmares
- Insomnia
- Constipation
- Dry mouth

Most common (>5% and at least twice the placebo rate) as adjunct therapy
to psychostimulants in ADHD in 6- to 17-year-olds are

■ Somnolence
■ Fatigue
■ Decreased appetite
■ Dizziness

*Drug interactions* include

■ Sedating drugs (alcohol, barbiturates, others)
■ Tricyclic antidepressants (may reduce hypotensive effect of clonidine)
■ Drugs known to affect sinus node function or atrioventricular node
  conduction (eg, digitalis, calcium channel blocking agent, α-adrenergic
  blocking agent) because of potential additive, such as bradycardia and
  atrioventricular block
■ Antihypertensive drugs

## Vital Signs and Laboratory Monitoring

For all clonidine preparations, monitoring blood pressure and heart rate is
recommended. No specific laboratory studies are recommended.

## Optimizing Dose

A general recommendation for optimizing dose—if confident that the child
has adhered to the previously prescribed dose—is to continue to increase
the dose until the benefit-to-risk ratio is optimized. Treatment response,
assessed systematically using information from parent and teacher reports
(eg, NICHQ Vanderbilt Assessment Scale ratings), should be considered
alongside reported and observed adverse effects during dose escalation.
Satisfaction of the caregiver, teacher, and child regarding the child's response
can also be useful. Ideally, a consensus will emerge about the preferred dose
that maximizes the benefit-to-risk ratio.

Specifics regarding dosage adjustments were presented in the previous Dosage Adjustments section.

## Maintenance

Once an optimal dose is determined, maintenance treatment begins.
Frequency of monitoring can be reduced, usually to follow-ups every 1 to
3 months, depending on the patient's needs. Consideration of dose

adjustments is recommended annually, or more often, if the patient's clinical status changes significantly.

## What if a Clonidine Preparation Is Ineffective or Not Tolerated?

If adverse effects limit sufficient dose escalation or if the maximal recommended dose is not effective, discontinuation is recommended. If continued medication is clinically indicated, consideration of another class of ADHD medication may be warranted.

## Discontinuing Clonidine and Possible Withdrawal Adverse Effects

To minimize withdrawal adverse effects, it is recommended that ER clonidine be tapered in daily dose increments of 0.1 mg every 3 to 7 days. Blood pressure and pulse monitoring is recommended during taper and discontinuation.

Potential withdrawal adverse effects include rebound increases in blood pressure and heart rate.

## Switching From One to Another Clonidine Preparation

The following text is taken verbatim from the Kapvay package insert[13(p3)]: "Due to lack of controlled clinical trial data and differing pharmacokinetic profiles, substitution of Kapvay for other clonidine products on a mg-per-mg basis is not recommended." Thus, cross-tapering should be done cautiously.

## Adjunct Treatment to Stimulants

Extended-release clonidine is FDA approved for adjunctive treatment to stimulants. This may be considered when the stimulant dose cannot be optimized because of adverse effects in the context of persisting ADHD symptoms. Recommendations for using adjunctive clonidine preparations are the same as when it is used alone. It is important to note that combination treatment may be prone to a higher likelihood of adverse effects and that, in general, treatment with one medication is preferable, when possible.

## When to Consult or Refer

In general, consultation with, or referral to, a child and adolescent psychiatrist or other prescribing specialist may be considered when there is lack of clarity about diagnosis or after several medications have been tried and discontinued because of lack of effect or tolerability. A more extensive discussion regarding what to do when interventions fail is presented in Chapter 8.

# Atomoxetine

## Available Atomoxetine Preparations

Atomoxetine is a selective norepinephrine reuptake inhibitor. Atomoxetine is available in the United States as Strattera. A generic atomoxetine is not available.

Atomoxetine has a therapeutic effect on ADHD symptoms comparable to that of guanfacine and clonidine but less than the stimulants. Much of the information in this section is from the Strattera package insert.[14]

## Onset of Effect

The time to initial and full effect of atomoxetine is much longer than for stimulants and $\alpha_2$-adrenergic agonists: about 1 to 2 *weeks* for initial effect and 4 to 6 weeks for full effect. Families should be advised of this delayed response so they don't discontinue treatment prematurely.

## Duration of Effect

Once atomoxetine reaches peak effect after about 2 to 4 weeks on a stable therapeutic dose, its therapeutic effect is continuous.

## Initial Dose

*Up to 70 kg body weight:* 0.5 mg/kg/day in the morning or in 2 divided doses.

*More than 70 kg body weight:* 40 mg/day in the morning or in 2 divided doses.

## Dosage Adjustments

*Up to 70 kg body weight:* After a minimum of 3 days on the initial dose, atomoxetine can be increased to a target daily dose of approximately 1.2 mg/kg, administered as a single daily dose or as evenly divided doses in the morning and late afternoon or evening. No additional benefit has been demonstrated for doses greater than 1.2 mg/kg/day, although the maximum daily dose is listed as 1.4 mg/kg/day or 100 mg/day, whichever is less.

*More than 70 kg body weight:* After a minimum of 3 days on the initial dose, atomoxetine can be increased to a target daily dose of approximately 80 mg, administered as a single daily dose or as evenly divided doses in the morning and late afternoon or evening. After 2 to 4 additional weeks, the total daily dose may be increased to a total daily dose of 100 mg in patients who have not achieved an optimal response. No additional benefit has been demonstrated for higher doses.

## Monitoring Therapeutic Response During Dose Adjustments

During dose adjustment, a weekly phone check-in or appointment is preferred. Parent and teacher NICHQ Vanderbilt Assessment Scale reports can facilitate tracking change in severity of symptoms.

## Safety Monitoring

Monitoring for contraindications, adverse effects, and potential drug interactions starts before medication is prescribed and continues throughout drug administration. As with all medications, safety monitoring for atomoxetine depends on a targeted history and physical examination. The information below is based on the package insert for Strattera.[14] Safety data for this package insert is derived, in part, from clinical trials involving youth, aged 6 to 17.

### Contraindications

- Hypersensitivity to atomoxetine or other constituents of the product
- Atomoxetine use within 2 weeks after discontinuing an MAOI or other drugs that affect brain monoamine concentrations
- Narrow angle glaucoma
- Pheochromocytoma or history of pheochromocytoma
- Severe cardiovascular disorders that may deteriorate with clinically important increases in heart rate or blood pressure

*Boxed warning:* Suicidal ideation.

### Warnings and precautions

- *Suicidal ideation:* Monitor for suicidal ideation, clinical worsening, and unusual changes in behavior.
- *Severe liver injury:* Should be discontinued and not restarted in patients with jaundice or laboratory evidence of liver injury.
- *Serious cardiovascular events:* Sudden death, stroke, and myocardial infarction have been reported in association with atomoxetine treatment. Patients should have a careful history and physical examination to access for presence of cardiovascular disease. Strattera generally should not be used in children or adolescents with known serious structural cardiac

abnormalities, cardiomyopathy, serious heart rhythm abnormalities, or other serious cardiac problems that may place them at increased vulnerability to its noradrenergic events.

- *Emergent cardiovascular symptoms:* Patients should undergo prompt cardiac evaluation.
- *Effects on blood pressure and heart rate:* Increase in blood pressure and heart rate, orthostasis, and syncope may occur. Use with caution in patients with hypertension, tachycardia, or cardiovascular or cerebrovascular disease.
- *Emergent psychotic or manic symptoms:* Consider discontinuing treatment if such new symptoms occur.
- *Bipolar disorder:* Screen patients to avoid possible induction of a mixed or manic episode.
- *Aggressive behavior or hostility:* Should be monitored.
- *Possible allergic reactions:* Including anaphylactic reactions, angioneurotic edema, urticarial, and rash.
- *Effects on urine outflow:* Urinary retention and hesitancy may occur.
- *Priapism:* Prompt medical attention is required in the event of suspected priapism.
- *Growth:* Height and weight should be monitored in pediatric patients.
- *Concomitant use of potent CYP2D6 inhibitors (eg, fluoxetine, paroxetine, quinidine):* Dose adjustment may be necessary.
- *Use in patients known to be CYP2D6 poor metabolizers:* Dose adjustment may be necessary.

**Adverse reactions:** Most common (>5% and at least twice the placebo rate) in child and adolescent trials of ADHD (6- to 17-year-olds) are

- Nausea
- Vomiting
- Fatigue
- Decreased appetite
- Abdominal pain
- Somnolence

**Drug interactions** include

- Monoamine oxidase inhibitors
- CYP2D6 inhibitors (Concomitant use may increase atomoxetine steady-state plasma concentrations in extensive metabolizers.)
- Antihypertensive drugs and pressor agents (possible effects on blood pressure)

■ Albuterol or other $\beta_2$-adrenergic agonists (Action of albuterol on the cardiovascular system can be potentiated.)

## Vital Signs and Laboratory Monitoring

Monitoring blood pressure, heart rate, height, and weight is recommended. No specific laboratory studies are recommended.

## Optimizing Dose

A general recommendation for optimizing dose—if confident that the child has adhered to the previously prescribed dose—is to continue to increase the dose until the benefit-to-risk ratio is optimized. Treatment response, assessed systematically using information from parent and teacher reports (eg, NICHQ Vanderbilt Assessment Scale ratings), should be considered alongside reported and observed adverse effects during dose escalation. Satisfaction of the caregiver, teacher, and child regarding the child's response can also be useful. Ideally, a consensus will emerge about the preferred dose that maximizes the benefit-to-risk ratio.

Specifics regarding dosage adjustments are presented in the previous Dosage Adjustments section.

## Maintenance

Once an optimal dose is determined, maintenance treatment begins. Frequency of monitoring can be reduced, usually to follow-ups every 1 to 3 months, depending on the patient's needs. Consideration of dose adjustments is recommended annually, or more often, if the patient's clinical status changes significantly.

## What if Atomoxetine Is Ineffective or Not Tolerated?

If adverse effects limit sufficient dose escalation or if the maximal recommended dose is not effective, discontinuation is recommended. If continued medication is clinically indicated, consideration of another class of ADHD medication may be warranted.

## Discontinuing Atomoxetine

Atomoxetine can be discontinued without tapering. There are no reported withdrawal-induced adverse effects.

## Adjunct Treatment to Stimulants

There is limited information regarding concomitant use of a stimulant and atomoxetine, although no data indicate a problem with this combination. The only relevant comment in the Strattera package insert is in Section 7.7: "Co-administration of methylphenidate with Strattera did not increase cardiovascular effects beyond those seen with methylphenidate alone."[14]

Adjunctive treatment may be considered when the stimulant dose cannot be optimized because of adverse effects yet clinically impairing ADHD symptoms persist. Recommendations for using adjunctive atomoxetine are the same as when it is used alone. It is important to note that combination treatment may be prone to a higher likelihood of adverse effects and that, in general, treatment with one medication is preferable, when possible.

## When to Consult or Refer

In general, consultation with, or referral to, a child and adolescent psychiatrist or other prescribing specialist may be considered when there is lack of clarity about diagnosis or after several medications have been tried and discontinued because of lack of effect or tolerability. A more extensive discussion regarding what to do when interventions fail is presented in Chapter 8.

# Summary

Five medications—the stimulants methylphenidate and amphetamine, the $\alpha_2$-adrenergic agonists guanfacine and clonidine, and the selective norepinephrine inhibitor atomoxetine—are FDA approved for treatment of ADHD in children and adolescents. It is recommended that pediatric PCCs develop familiarity with these medication groups to provide safe, effective, evidence-based pharmacologic treatment to children with ADHD.

American Academy of Pediatrics and American Academy of Child Adolescent and Psychiatry guidelines and practice parameters suggest starting treatment with one of the stimulants. There are multiple available preparations of methylphenidate and amphetamine, with the major difference between these being their duration of effect. It is recommended that pediatric PCCs develop familiarity with stimulant preparations with various durations of effect. Available data suggest that a methylphenidate or an amphetamine preparation is effective in almost all children, so switching from one to the other is generally indicated if the first is not effective.

Guanfacine, clonidine, and atomoxetine are secondary options, with lower effectiveness than stimulants; they can be used independently or as adjunctive treatment if stimulants cannot be tolerated or are only partially or not effective. An advantage of guanfacine over clonidine is once-daily dosing in contrast to twice-daily dosing with clonidine. In contrast to the stimulants and $\alpha_2$-adrenergic agonists, atomoxetine has a much delayed onset of effect (about 4–6 weeks).

Medication should be part of a comprehensive treatment plan that includes, when indicated, appropriate behavior therapy(ies) and school consultation.

# References

1. Visser SN, Bitsko RH, Danielson ML, et al. Treatment of attention deficit/hyperactivity disorder among children with special health care needs. *J Pediatr.* 2015;166(6): 1423–1430
2. American Academy of Pediatrics Subcommittee on Attention-Deficit/Hyperactivity Disorder, Steering Committee on Quality Improvement; Wolraich M, Brown L, Brown RT, et al. ADHD: clinical practice guideline for the diagnosis, evaluation, and treatment of attention-deficit/hyperactivity disorder in children and adolescents. *Pediatrics.* 2011;128(5):1007–1022
3. Pliszka S, AACAP Work Group on Quality Issues. Practice parameter for the assessment and treatment of children and adolescents with attention-deficit/hyperactivity disorder. *J Am Acad Child Adolesc Psychiatry.* 2007;46(7):894–921
4. Greenhill L, Kollins S, Abikoff H, et al. Efficacy and safety of immediate-release methylphenidate treatment for preschoolers with ADHD. *J Am Acad Child Adolesc Psychiatry.* 2007;45(11):1284–1293
5. Gleason MM, Egger HL, Emslie GJ, et al. Psychopharmacological treatment for very young children: contexts and guidelines. *J Am Acad Child Adolesc Psychiatry.* 2007;46(12):1532–1572
6. Riddle MA, Yershova K, Lazzaretto D, et al. The Preschool Attention-Deficit/Hyperactivity Disorder Treatment Study (PATS) 6-year follow-up. *J Am Acad Child Adolesc Psychiatry.* 2013;52(3):264–278
7. Wilson JJ. ADHD and substance use disorders: developmental aspects and the impact of stimulant treatment. *Am J Addict.* 2007;16(Suppl 1):5–11
8. Biederman J, Monuteaux MC, Spencer T, Wilens TE, Macpherson HA, Faraone SV. Stimulant therapy and risk for subsequent substance use disorders in male adults with ADHD: a naturalistic controlled 10-year follow-up study. *Am J Psychiatry.* 2008;165(5):597–603
9. Mannuzza S, Klein RG, Troung NL, et al. Age of methylphenidate treatment initiation with ADHD and later substance abuse: prospective follow-up into adulthood. *Am J Psychiatry.* 2008;165(5):604–609
10. Wilens TE, Adler LA, Adams J, et al. Misuse and diversion of stimulants prescribed for ADHD: a systematic review of the literature. *J Am Acad Child Adolesc Psychiatry.* 2008;47(1):21–31

11. Perrin JM, Friedman RA, Knilans TK; American Academy of Pediatrics Black Box Working Group, Section on Cardiology and Cardiac Surgery. Cardiovascular monitoring and stimulant drugs for attention-deficit/hyperactivity disorder. *Pediatrics.* 2008;122(2):451–453
12. Intuniv [package insert]. FDA Web site. http://www.fda.gov. Accessed July 15, 2015
13. Kapvay [package insert]. FDA Web site. http://www.fda.gov. Accessed July 15, 2015
14. Strattera [package insert]. FDA Web site. http://www.fda.gov. Accessed July 15, 2015

# CHAPTER 5

# Group 1 Medications for Anxiety and Depression

## General Guidance

### Medications

Recommendations for pharmacologic treatment of depression are straightforward: fluoxetine and escitalopram have US Food and Drug Administration (FDA) indications for treatment of major depressive disorder (MDD) in youth.

Recommendations for pharmacologic treatment of anxiety have a more complex rationale. The FDA has not approved medication for treatment of any anxiety disorder in youth, other than obsessive-compulsive disorder (OCD), an anxiety-like disorder. (See Evidence Supporting Efficacy section in Chapter 1 for an explanation of technical reasons.) However, there have been high-quality, National Institutes of Health (NIH)–sponsored, multisite studies demonstrating effectiveness of fluoxetine, sertraline, and fluvoxamine for the 3 common anxiety disorders in youth: generalized anxiety disorder, social anxiety disorder, and separation anxiety disorder. These 3 selective serotonin reuptake inhibitors (SSRIs) have FDA indications for use in youth with OCD (as well as various anxiety disorders in adults) and are recommended for treatment of common anxiety disorders in youth.

Throughout this chapter, the 4 SSRIs will be treated the same, unless specifically noted when differences are worthy of comment.

The 4 SSRIs in Group 1 that are recommended for treatment of anxiety or depression are presented in Table 5.1.

**Table 5.1. Group 1 Selective Serotonin Reuptake Inhibitors for Anxiety and Depression**

| Generic Name | Trade Name | US FDA Youth Indication(s), years | Initial Dose, mg | Max DD, mg | Dosing Frequency | Available Unit Dose Forms |
|---|---|---|---|---|---|---|
| Fluoxetine | Prozac | MDD; 8–17<br>OCD; 7–17 | 10–20 (5–10[a]) | 60 | Daily | Capsules: 10, 20, and 40 mg<br>Weekly capsules: 90 mg |
| Escitalopram | Lexapro | MDD; 12–17 | 10 mg (5–10[a]) | 20 | Daily | Tablets: 5, 10 (scored), and 20 (scored) mg<br>Oral solution: 1 mg/mL |
| Sertraline | Zoloft | OCD; 6–17 | 6–12 years: 25<br>13–17 years: 50 | 200 | Daily | Scored tablets: 25, 50, and 100 mg<br>Oral solution: 20 mg/mL |
| Fluvoxamine | NA in United States | OCD; 8–17 | 25 | 8–11 years: 200<br>12–17 years: 300 | Twice a day[b] | Tablets: 25, 50, and 100 mg |

Abbreviations: FDA, Food and Drug Administration; Max DD, maximum recommended daily dose based on FDA-approved package insert; MDD, major depressive disorder; OCD, obsessive-compulsive disorder; NA, not available.

[a] Author's recommendation.

[b] Divided doses (twice a day) if total daily dose is over 50 mg.

Classified using US Food and Drug Administration. Drugs@FDA Web site. http://www.accessdata.fda.gov/scripts/cder/drugsatfda. Accessed July 15, 2015.

## Reminder About Psychosocial Interventions

Evidence-based and effective psychotherapies for youth with anxiety or depression are considered first-line treatment; these are discussed in detail in the Psychosocial Treatments section in Chapter 3. Cognitive-behavioral therapy (CBT), with a caregiver and family component, is the most effective psychotherapy for youth with anxiety. Cognitive behavioral therapy and interpersonal psychotherapy (IPT) are the most effective psychotherapies for youth with depression. A substantial body of evidence indicates that combining psychotherapy with medication can enhance effectiveness of medication.

## Choosing a Medication

No guidance regarding selection of a specific SSRI is available from the American Academy of Pediatrics or American Academy of Child and Adolescent Psychiatry.

For depression, SSRIs with FDA approval for treatment of MDD in youth are preferred (ie, fluoxetine and escitalopram). For anxiety, SSRIs with FDA approval for treatment of OCD in youth, and supporting efficacy and safety data for the common anxiety disorders in youth, are preferred (ie, fluoxetine, sertraline, and fluvoxamine).

Other issues that may influence selection of an SSRI include half-life, once-daily dosing, and potential drug-drug interactions. Fluoxetine, which has a much longer half-life (days to weeks) than other SSRIs, may be advantageous for patients with sporadic adherence. Fluvoxamine may be less convenient than other SSRIs because it needs to be taken twice a day, in contrast with other SSRIs that can be dosed once a day. Escitalopram may be advantageous when there are concerns about drug-drug interactions because it has the least effect on CYP450 isoenzymes compared with other SSRIs.

## Adverse Effects, Contraindications, and Drug Interactions

Adverse effects can be evaluated based on either severity or frequency. In package inserts required by the FDA, potential severity of adverse effects is emphasized; that is, Boxed Warnings are more severe than Warnings and Precautions, which are more severe than Adverse Reactions. In addition, package inserts describe Contraindications and Drug Interactions.

The most comprehensive and least potentially biased prescribing information about adverse effects can be found in FDA-required package inserts. These inserts are available in various formats and locations, including in medication packaging and the *Physician's Desk Reference*. They are available online at Drugs@FDA, where they are referred to as labels. Since the FDA modified the format for package inserts a few years ago, each one has a one-page *Highlights of Prescribing Information* that includes relatively complete and essential information about boxed warnings, warnings and precautions, adverse effects, contraindications, and drug interactions. These highlights can be accessed and reviewed quickly and conveniently and are recommended as useful resources.

## Cost and Affordability

Generic medications are available for all 4 Group 1 SSRIs and are typically less expensive than brand medication. Please refer to the Cost and Affordability section in Chapter 4 for a discussion of cost and affordability of psychotropic medications.

## Information for Caregivers About Specific Medications

There are numerous sources of information about medications for patients, parents, and caregivers(s), particularly on various Web sites. Many, if not all, of these sources are supported, at least in part, by funds from the pharmaceutical industry. Potentially the least biased source is the FDA. At the end of each package insert (available online at Drugs@FDA) is a user-friendly document entitled *Medication Guide* or *Patient Counseling and Information*. This document should be given to the patient (or caregiver) by the dispensing pharmacist (including mail-order pharmacies). In addition, the prescribing clinician can print the document and go over it with the caregiver or patient.

# Group 1 Selective Serotonin Reuptake Inhibitors

## Available SSRI Preparations

Group 1 SSRIs—fluoxetine, escitalopram, sertraline, and fluvoxamine—are listed in Table 5.1 along with

- Trade name
- FDA indications in youth
- Recommended initial dose
- Recommended maximum dose
- Dosing frequency
- Available unit dose forms of each medication

Information in the table relies on FDA-approved package inserts or, occasionally, the author's recommendation when specific information is not available.

## Initial Dose

Table 5.1 presents recommended initial dose for each SSRI. In general, the younger the patient, the smaller the recommended initial dose. Prepubertal children are particularly sensitive to hyperkinesis, insomnia, and restlessness (sometimes called "activation"), and these adverse effects appear to be dose responsive.

## Onset of Effect

Onset of effect for all Group 1 SSRIs generally occurs after 3 to 4 weeks at an effective dose. This 3- to 4-week delay is not from the time of initial dose but from the time of effective dose, which may occur several weeks after initial dose, depending on speed and extent of dose titration. Onset of some adverse effects, such as abdominal pain or discomfort, can occur within days of the initial dose and may worsen during dose titration. In addition, some therapeutic effects, such as improved sleep, may occur before more global improvement in anxiety or depression symptoms.

## Duration of Effect

The effect of SSRIs is continuous as long as the medication is taken as recommended.

## Dosage Adjustments

Dosage adjustment for SSRIs requires balancing desire to reach a therapeutic dose as quickly as possible with reality that an effect of a dose change may not be observable for 2 to 4 weeks. A practical approach to dose escalation that balances this desire and reality is to increase the dose every 4 to 7 days by an amount approximately equivalent to the starting dose while observing for adverse effects. If no or minimal adverse effects occur, dose increases may continue, as long as there is consistent communication between the patient and pediatric primary care clinician (pediatric PCC) and the pediatric PCC is confident of adherence. Dose increases can be delayed or reversed, depending on the clinical situation. Gastrointestinal and activation adverse effects may resolve spontaneously if dose escalation is slowed temporarily. This process can be continued until an optimal dose or the recommended maximum daily dose is reached.

## Monitoring Therapeutic Response During Dose Adjustments

During dose adjustment, a weekly phone check-in or appointment is preferred, when possible. Standardized rating scales, such as the Screen for Anxiety Related Disorders (SCARED) for anxiety and Patient Health Questionnaire-9 (PHQ-9) Modified for Teens for depression, may be helpful in systematically assessing symptom change (see Appendix A). Recommended safety monitoring is described in the next 2 sections.

## Safety Monitoring

Monitoring for contraindications, adverse effects, and potential drug interactions starts before medication is prescribed and continues throughout drug administration. As with all medications, safety monitoring for SSRIs depends on a targeted history and physical examination. The information below is derived from FDA-approved package inserts for the 4 Group 1 SSRIs.

*Contraindications* include

- Known hypersensitivity (*escitalopram and sertraline only*).
- Serotonin syndrome and monoamine oxidase inhibitors (MAOIs) (*all 4 Group 1 SSRIs*).
  - Do not use SSRIs and MAOIs concomitantly.
  - Do not start SSRI within 14 days of stopping MAOI (*escitalopram, fluvoxamine, sertraline*).
  - Do not start SSRI within 5 weeks of stopping MAOI (*fluoxetine*).
- Pimozide: Do not use concomitantly (*all 4 Group 1 SSRIs*).
- Thioridazine: Do not use concomitantly (*fluoxetine and fluvoxamine only*).
- Coadministration of tizanidine or alosetron (*fluvoxamine only*).

*Boxed warnings* include suicidal thoughts and behaviors (*all 4 Group 1 SSRIs*). Monitor for worsening or emergence of suicidal thoughts and behaviors.

*Warnings and precautions:* Most warnings and precautions are relatively rare in children and adolescents treated with SSRIs. Warnings and precautions are listed below. Those in the package insert of all 4 Group 1 SSRIs are at the top; those for just one SSRI are at the bottom. Below each warning or precaution are recommendations for monitoring.

- *Clinical worsening and suicide risk (all 4 Group 1 SSRIs).* Monitor for clinical worsening and suicidal thinking and behavior.

- *Serotonin syndrome (all 4 Group 1 SSRIs).* Avoid administering or monitor carefully when coadministering other serotonergic agents, including triptans, tricyclic antidepressants, fentanyl, lithium, tramadol, tryptophan, buspirone, and St. John's wort.
- *Activation of mania or hypomania (all 4 Group 1 SSRIs).* Screen for bipolar disorder and monitor for mania or hypomania.
- *Seizures (all 4 Group 1 SSRIs).* Use cautiously in patients with a history of seizures or with conditions that potentially lower the seizure threshold.
- *Abnormal bleeding (all 4 Group 1 SSRIs).* Use with nonsteroidal anti-inflammatory drugs, aspirin, warfarin, or other drugs that affect coagulation may potentiate the risk of gastrointestinal or other bleeding.
- *Angle-closure glaucoma (all 4 Group 1 SSRIs).* Avoid administering to patients with known and untreated anatomically narrow angles.
- *Hyponatremia (all 4 Group 1 SSRIs).* Consider discontinuing if symptomatic hyponatremia occurs (eg, in patients with syndrome of inappropriate antidiuretic hormone).
- *Potential for cognitive and motor impairment (fluoxetine, escitalopram, sertraline).* Advise using caution when operating machinery.
- *Discontinuation of treatment (escitalopram, sertraline, fluvoxamine).* A gradual reduction in dose rather than abrupt cessation is recommended whenever possible.
- *Use in patients with concomitant illness (escitalopram, sertraline, fluvoxamine).* Use caution in patients with diseases or conditions that produce altered metabolism or hemodynamic reactions.
- *Altered appetite, weight, or both (fluoxetine, sertraline).* Monitor weight, primarily for potential weight loss.
- *Allergic reactions and rash (fluoxetine).* Discontinue on appearance of rash or allergic phenomena.
- *Anxiety and insomnia (fluoxetine).* Be aware that these reactions may occur.
- *QT prolongation (fluoxetine).* Use caution in conditions that predispose to arrhythmias or increased fluoxetine exposure. Use cautiously in patients with risk factors for QT prolongation.
- *Long half-life (fluoxetine).* Be aware that changes in dose will not be reflected in plasma for several weeks.
- *Other potentially important drug interactions (fluvoxamine).* Coadministration with a benzodiazepine is generally not advisable. Use with caution in patients taking clozapine, methadone, mexiletine, ramelteon, theophylline, or warfarin.

*Adverse reactions:* Across the package inserts for the 4 Group 1 SSRIs is considerable consistency, and some variability, in adverse effects listed. All 4 package inserts list the most common reactions in adults observed in placebo-controlled clinical trials with an incidence greater than or equal to 5% and an incidence at least twice that for placebo. The package inserts also state that adverse effects observed in pediatric studies were similar to those in adult studies. Data from relatively small numbers of pediatric study participants are also presented. The most consistently reported adverse effects are listed below. More details may be found in the specific package insert for each SSRI.

- Nausea
- Diarrhea and loose stools
- Insomnia
- Somnolence
- Fatigue
- Sexual (decreased libido, anorgasmia, ejaculatory delay)
- Sweating increased
- Agitation or hyperkinesis
- Tremor

*Drug interactions:* Drug interactions listed in package inserts vary across the 4 Group 1 SSRIs and, in many instances, overlap with warnings and precautions. The most salient drug interactions are listed below. More details may be found in the specific package insert for each SSRI.

- SSRIs, serotonin-norepinephrine reuptake inhibitors, or tryptophan
- Drugs that affect homeostasis (nonsteroidal anti-inflammatory drugs, aspirin, warfarin)
- MAOIs
- Drugs that prolong the QT interval (eg, pimozide or thioridazine)
- *For fluoxetine and sertraline:* drugs metabolized by CYP2D6
- *For fluvoxamine:* drugs inhibiting or metabolized by CYP1A2, CYP2C9, CYP3A4 and CYP2C19

## Vital Signs and Laboratory Monitoring

For all SSRIs, monitoring height and weight is recommended. No specific laboratory studies are recommended.

## Optimizing Dose

A general recommendation for optimizing dose—if confident that the child has adhered to the previously prescribed dose—is to continue to increase the dose until the benefit-to-risk ratio is optimized. Treatment response, assessed systematically using information from the parent and the patient's self-reports (eg, SCARED for anxiety and PHQ-9 Modified for Teens for depression) should be considered alongside reported and observed adverse effects during dose escalation. The caregiver's and child's satisfaction with the child's response can also be useful. Ideally, a consensus will emerge about the preferred dose that maximizes the benefit-to-risk ratio.

## Maintenance

Once an optimal dose is determined, maintenance treatment begins. Frequency of monitoring can be reduced, usually to follow-ups every 1 to 3 months, depending on the patient's needs. Consider dose adjustments annually, or more often, if the patient's clinical status changes significantly.

## What if the First SSRI Is Ineffective or Not Tolerated?

If adverse effects limit sufficient dose escalation or if the initial SSRI is not considered sufficiently beneficial, consider discontinuation of SSRI.

## Discontinuing an SSRI and Possible Withdrawal Adverse Effects

To minimize withdrawal adverse effects, a gradual reduction in dose over a few weeks, rather than abrupt discontinuation, is recommended, except for fluoxetine. Because of fluoxetine's (and its active metabolite's) long half-life, it can be discontinued abruptly and will "self-taper." Withdrawal adverse effects, particularly with abrupt discontinuation, may include dysphoric mood, irritability, agitation, insomnia, anxiety, headache, emotional lability, and flu-like symptoms.

## Switching From One to Another SSRI

The best available research indicates that for depression in adolescents if the initial SSRI "fails," the next-best medication option is another SSRI.[1]

Switching from one SSRI to another can be staggered and overlapping, as long as the combined total daily dose remains equivalent and comparable. A staggered switch can usually be completed over a few weeks. If fluoxetine is discontinued abruptly, dose escalation of the new SSRI can be based on an approximate half-life of fluoxetine of 1 to 2 weeks.

## When to Consult or Refer

In general, consultation with, or referral to, a child and adolescent psychiatrist or other prescribing specialist may be considered when there is lack of clarity about diagnosis or after several medications have been tried and discontinued because of lack of effect or tolerability. A more extensive discussion regarding what to do when interventions fail is presented in Chapter 8.

# Summary

Four Group 1 SSRIs are recommended for treatment of anxiety or depression. No guidance regarding selection of a specific SSRI is available from the American Academy of Pediatrics or the American Academy of Child Adolescent Psychiatry. For depression, SSRIs with FDA approval for treatment of MDD in youth are preferred: fluoxetine and escitalopram. For anxiety, SSRIs with FDA approval for treatment of OCD in youth, and supporting efficacy and safety data for common anxiety disorders, are preferred: fluoxetine, sertraline, and fluvoxamine.

Other parameters that may influence selection of an SSRI include half-life, once-daily dosing, and potential drug-drug interactions. Fluoxetine has a much longer half-life (days to weeks) than other SSRIs, which may be advantageous for patients with sporadic adherence. Fluvoxamine may be less convenient than other SSRIs because it needs to be taken twice a day in contrast with other SSRIs, which can be dosed once a day. Escitalopram may be advantageous when there are concerns about drug-drug interactions because it has the least effect on CYP450 isoenzymes compared with other SSRIs.

Medication should be part of a comprehensive treatment plan that includes, when indicated and available, evidence-based psychotherapy(ies).

# Reference

1. Brent D, Emslie G, Clark G, et al. Switching to another SSRI or to venlafaxine with or without cognitive behavioral therapy for adolescents with SSRI-resistant depression: the TORDIA randomized control trial. *JAMA*. 2008;299(8):901–913

# Part 4—Group 2 (FDA-Approved Antipsychotics and Mood Stabilizers) and Group 3 (All Other) Medications

# CHAPTER 6

# Group 2 Medications: Antipsychotics and Mood Stabilizer

## Rationale

In addition to prescribing and monitoring Group 1 medications, pediatric primary care clinicians (pediatric PCCs) are ideally suited to collaborate with psychiatrists and other mental health specialists in the care of children with more severe or uncommon disorders. Thus, they may be asked to take on partial responsibility for monitoring therapeutic and adverse effects of a variety of other medications that are included in Groups 2 and 3.

Group 2 medications can be monitored in primary care settings, but, because they generally have a more concerning safety profile, more complicated monitoring requirements than Group 1 medications, or both, they are generally prescribed by specialists.

- Child psychiatrists
- Developmental-behavioral pediatricians
- Specialists in neurodevelopmental disabilities or adolescent medicine
- Pediatric neurologists
- Adult psychiatrists with additional training in adolescent psychiatry

Depending on an individual pediatric PCC's skills and experience, and a lack of available of specialists for referral (especially in rural and underserved areas), some pediatric PCCs with additional training in pediatric psycho-pharmacology may choose to prescribe Group 2 medications.

Group 2 includes all US Food and Drug Administration (FDA)–approved medications for youth with other disorders (ie, not ADHD, anxiety, or depression). Group 2 includes 5 second-generation antipsychotics (SGAs) (aripiprazole, olanzapine, quetiapine, risperidone and paliperidone) and lithium, a mood stabilizer.

All 5 SGAs are approved for treatment of youth with psychosis in schizophrenia; all except paliperidone are approved for mania in bipolar disorder;
and only risperidone and aripiprazole are approved for "irritability" in
autism. However, these medications are most commonly used off-label (ie,
outside FDA indications) in youth to treat behavioral problems, especially
aggression (see later in the chapter for details).

Lithium is FDA approved for treatment of acute mania in bipolar disorder.
Lithium is also used off-label to treat non-bipolar mood instability.

# Antipsychotics

Antipsychotics can be both beneficial and problematic. They are very
effective at reducing severity of a wide range of symptoms, but they are also
associated with a variety of major adverse effects.

## Effects, Indications, Ages, Equivalencies, and Dosages

Specific therapeutic effects of antipsychotics include

- Antipsychotic effects for hallucinations, delusions, and disorganized
  thinking
- Mood-stabilizing effects for mania, irritability, and mood instability
- Possible "organizing" or "calming" effects for agitation and aggressive
  behavior

The 10 SGAs available in the United States are presented in Table 6.1. The 5
that have an indication in children or adolescents, and, thus, are included in
Group 2, are noted.

Table 6.2 lists the indications by disorder and age range for the 5 SGAs on the
US market.

Table 6.3 lists drug equivalencies for the 5 FDA-approved SGAs, using
risperidone as the comparator with an equivalency of 1. Also included for
comparison are ziprasidone (Geodon), which is one of the Group 3 medications described in Chapter 7, and haloperidol, a traditional antipsychotic.
The equivalencies in Table 6.3 are based on the best available data.[1] These
data are based on the minimal necessary dose for treatment of psychosis in
schizophrenia in adults. No such comparative data are available for children and adolescents or for symptoms and disorders other than psychosis

**Table 6.1. Second-Generation Antipsychotics**

| Medication | Brand Name | Marketed Since |
|---|---|---|
| Clozapine | Clozaril | 1989 |
| Risperidone[a] | Risperdal | 1990s |
| Quetiapine[a] | Seroquel | 1990s |
| Aripiprazole[a] | Abilify | 1990s |
| Olanzapine[a] | Zyprexa | 1990s |
| Ziprasidone | Geodon | 1990s |
| Paliperidone[a] | Invega | 2006 |
| Iloperidone | Fanapt | 2006 |
| Asenapine | Saphris | 2006 |
| Lurasidone | Latuda | 2011 |

[a] US Food and Drug Administration approved for use in some youth younger than 18 years as of March 5, 2015.

**Table 6.2. SGAs and Pediatric US FDA Indications**

| Drug | Disorder | | |
|---|---|---|---|
| Risperidone | SCZ | BPM | ASD-I[a] |
| Aripiprazole | SCZ | BPM | ASD-I[a] |
| Quetiapine | SCZ | BPM | NA |
| Olanzapine | SCZ | BPM[b] | NA |
| Paliperidone | SCZ[c] | NA | NA |

Abbreviations: ASD-I, "irritability" in autism; BPM, mania in bipolar disorder; FDA, Food and Drug Administration; NA, not applicable; SCZ, psychosis in schizophrenia; SGA, second-generation antipsychotic.
Ages, years
[a] ASD-I = ≥5 for risperidone and ≥6 for aripiprazole.
[b] BPM = ≥10, except for olanzapine at ≥13.
[c] SCZ = ≥13, except for paliperidone at ≥12.
Classified using US Food and Drug Administration. Drugs@FDA Web site. http://www.accessdata.fda.gov/scripts/cder/drugsatfda/index.cfm. Accessed March 5, 2015.

in schizophrenia. Thus, these equivalencies are meant to serve as a general guide, not as a definitive conversion factor.

Table 6.4 lists initial, recommended, and maximal doses for various indicated disorders for the 5 FDA-approved SGAs. These doses were taken directly from the first page of the drug label for each drug at the Web site Drugs@FDA. Again, they are meant as guides, not only for clinicians who

**Table 6.3. Dose Equivalency of Selected Antipsychotic Medications[a]**

| Medication | Dose Equivalency, mg |
|---|---|
| Risperidone | 1 |
| Aripiprazole | 5 |
| Quetiapine | 75 |
| Olanzapine | 4 |
| Paliperidone | 1.5 |
| Ziprasidone | 20 |
| Haloperidol | 2 |

[a] Data from adults with schizophrenia; no data available in children and adolescents.

Classified using Leucht S, Samara M, Heres S, Patel MX, Woods SW, Davis JM. Dose equivalents for second-generation antipsychotics: the minimum effective dose method. *Schizophr Bull.* 2014;40(2):314–326.

**Table 6.4. US FDA-Recommended Dose for Group 2 SGAs in Youth**

| Medication | Indication | Ages, years | Initial Dose, mg | Recommended Dose, mg | Maximum Dose, mg |
|---|---|---|---|---|---|
| Risperidone | Psychosis in SCZ | 13–17 | 0.5 | 3[a] | 6[b] |
| | Mania in bipolar | 10–17 | 0.5 | 1.0–2.5[a] | 6[b] |
| | "Irritability" in autism | 5–17 | 0.25 (<20 kg) 0.5 (≥20 kg) | 0.5 (<20 kg)[a] 1.0 (≥20 kg)[a] | 3[b] 3[b] |
| Aripiprazole | Psychosis in SCZ | 13–17 | 2 | 10 | 30 |
| | Mania in bipolar | 10–17 | 2 | 10 | 30 |
| | Irritability in autism | 6–17 | 2 | 5–10 | 15 |
| Quetiapine | Psychosis in SCZ | 13–17 | 25 twice a day | 400–800 | 800 |
| | Mania in bipolar | 10–17 | 25 twice a day | 400–800 | 600 |
| Olanzapine | Psychosis in SCZ | 13–17 | 2.5–5 | 10 | NA |
| | Mania in bipolar | 13–17 | 2.5–5 | 10 | NA |
| Paliperidone | Psychosis in SCZ | 12–17 | 3 (<51 kg) 3 (>51 kg) | 3–6 (<51 kg) 3–12 (>51 kg) | 6 (<51 kg) 12 (>51 kg) |

Abbreviations: FDA, Food and Drug Administration; NA, not applicable; SCZ, psychosis in schizophrenia; SGA, second-generation antipsychotic.

[a] No recommended dose is listed; instead, use Target Dose.

[b] No maximum dose is listed; instead, use highest dose in Effective Dose Range.

Classified using US Food and Drug Administration. Drugs@FDA. http://www.accessdata.fda.gov/scripts/cder/drugsatfda/index.cfm. Accessed March 5, 2015.

are prescribing these medications but also for those who are participating in monitoring their appropriateness, effectiveness, adverse effects, and related laboratory measures.

## Adverse Effects and Monitoring

Of all psychotropic medications used in children and adolescents, SGAs generally have the most concerning adverse effects, including

- Sedation
- Weight gain
- Elevated glucose
- Insulin resistance
- Elevated triglyceride and cholesterol levels
- Irreversible involuntary movements (tardive dyskinesia)
- Gynecomastia
- Galactorrhea

*Three relatively common adverse effects* of SGAs are listed in Box 6.1. Also, for the 4 SGAs for which data are available, the frequency of each type of adverse effect is displayed from left (most common) to right (least common). Sedation and anticholinergic effects, such as dry mouth or constipation, can be troubling for both patients and their parents and can lead to reduced adherence to or discontinuation of medication. If problematic, these adverse effects can be reduced or alleviated by lowering dose (especially for sedation) or switching to an SGA further to the right in Box 6.1. Tremor, which is usually mild in youth taking clinically appropriate doses, may also be reduced or alleviated by lowering the dose or switching medication.

*Three types of major potential adverse effects* of SGAs are presented in Box 6.2. Many of the major adverse effects of SGAs—particularly weight gain,

---

**Box 6.1. Three Relatively Common Adverse Effects Associated With Group 2 SGAs**

**Sedation**
Olanzapine > quetiapine > risperidone ≥ aripiprazole.

**Anticholinergic** (eg, dry mouth, constipation)
Olanzapine > quetiapine > risperidone = aripiprazole.

**Tremor**
Generally mild and not impairing

Abbreviation: SGA, second-generation antipsychotic.

**Box 6.2. Three Major Potential Adverse Effects Associated With Group 2 SGAs**

**Weight Gain**
Olanzapine > quetiapine > risperidone > aripiprazole.

**Metabolic Abnormalities** (eg, elevated glucose, cholesterol, or triglyceride level)
- Similar sequence because metabolic effects are secondary to weight gain.
- In addition, olanzapine has direct hepatic effect.

**Persistent Involuntary Movements**
- Tardive dyskinesia.
- Transient dyskinesia (during drug withdrawal).
- Differences between medications are unclear because these are rare in children.

Abbreviation: SGA, second-generation antipsychotic.
Classified using Correll CU, Manu P, Olshanskiy V, Napolitano B, Kane JM, Malhotra AK. Cardiometabolic risk of second-generation antipsychotic medications during first-time use in children and adolescents. *JAMA.* 2009;302(16):1765–1773 and Correll CU, Sheridan EM, DelBello MP. Antipsychotic and mood stabilizer efficacy and tolerability in pediatric and adult patients with bipolar I mania: a comparative analysis of acute, randomized, placebo-controlled trials. *Bipolar Disord.* 2010;12(2):116–14.

metabolic abnormalities, and delayed involuntary movements—can develop into major health problems (eg, cardiovascular disease and its consequences, tardive dyskinesia) during long-term treatment and may not be reversible.

There are individual differences in vulnerability to weight gain and the effect of metabolic changes. Some children will experience minimal if any weight or metabolic changes, while others may experience substantial increases in weight or changes in metabolism, even in response to treatment with relatively low doses.

Most disorders that are to be treated with SGAs are chronic and generally require long-term treatment. Thus, determining risk versus benefit of SGAs, both before and during ongoing treatment, is difficult and needs to be continuously evaluated.

*Box 6.3 presents 3 other important adverse effects or laboratory findings* associated with SGAs. Acute dystonia is relatively rare in children and occurs almost exclusively during the first few days of treatment or soon after an increase of dose. Acute dystonia can be quickly and effectively treated with benztropine or diphenhydramine. Once a child or adolescent is on a stable dose of an SGA, acute dystonia is very rare. Gynecomastia and galactorrhea are relatively uncommon and may be alleviated by lowering dosage or switching medications. Salivary hypersecretion and associated drooling can be very annoying to patients and may be alleviated by lowering dosage or switching medications. It appears to be more common with risperidone.

**Box 6.3. Three Other Important Adverse Events Associated With Group 2 SGAs**

| |
|---|
| **Acute Dystonia**<br>Unclear differences between medications |
| **Gynecomastia, Galactorrhea, or Both**<br>More commonly associated with risperidone; may be related to elevated prolactin level |
| **Salivary Hypersecretion and Drooling**<br>More commonly associated with risperidone; generally concerning to patients |

Abbreviation: SGA, second-generation antipsychotic.

*Severity of adverse effects* associated with SGAs can vary depending on the medication selected, dose, and duration of treatment (Box 6.4).

**Box 6.4. Treatment Variables That Can Intensify Severity of Adverse Effects**

| |
|---|
| **Drug**<br>SGAs vary regarding severity of various adverse effects (see Boxes 6.1, 6.2, and 6.3). |
| **Duration of SGA Treatment**<br>Longer-term exposure is generally associated with more weight increase, metabolic adverse effects, and possible tardive dyskinesia. |
| **Dose**<br>• Particularly relevant to weight-related and metabolic adverse effects.<br>• Only replicated data available is for risperidone. |

Abbreviations: SGA, second-generation antipsychotic.

*Monitoring for adverse effects of SGAs* includes a targeted history and physical examination and a few laboratory studies (see Box 6.5). There is no formal, widely-accepted protocol that specifies the content and frequency of monitoring in youth receiving SGAs. Monitoring at baseline, 12 weeks, 12 months, and then annually is a general (minimal) suggestion, that hopefully will be supported by (or need to be modified by) outcome data as more research results become available.

Management of individual adverse effects often starts with lowering dose or changing medication. Further evaluation by a specialist may be indicated (eg, gynecomastia, diabetes mellitus). Additional interventions are generally not medication specific and call on general medical management skills. For more detailed information, the "Practice Parameters for the Use of Atypical Antipsychotic Medications in Children and Adolescents" (available at www.aacap.org) is the only available formal guidance from the American Academy of Pediatrics or American Academy of Child and Adolescent Psychiatry for monitoring and treating adverse effects of SGAs.

**Box 6.5. Monitoring SGA Adverse Effects[a]**

| |
|---|
| **Sedation**<br>History and physical examination |
| **Gynecomastia, Galactorrhea, or Both**<br>History and physical examination (if positive, prolactin level) |
| **Anticholinergic** (eg, dry mouth, constipation)<br>History and physical examination |
| **Neurologic**<br>History and physical examination (including Abnormal Involuntary Movement Scale<br>[AIMS] and Barnes Akathisia Rating Scale) |
| **Other**<br>Hepatic function (ALT, AST, alkaline phosphatase)<br>Cardiac (baseline ECG for ziprasidone or for any SGA if significant cardiac history) |

Abbreviations: ECG, electrocardiogram; ALT, alanine transaminase; AST, aspartate transaminase; SGA, second-generation antipsychotic.

[a] Excluding weight-related and metabolic effects.

*Weight and potential metabolic adverse effects also need to be monitored.* The only available formal published guidance is for adults (Table 6.5). These published adult guidelines serve as a general framework for pediatric practice and are endorsed in the American Academy of Child and Adolescent Psychiatry practice parameters. The American Academy of Pediatrics has not issued formal guidelines or recommendations for monitoring antipsychotics.

A recently published survey[2] of prescribers of antipsychotics to patients younger than 18 years that used Vermont Medicaid data found that "physicians follow 'best practice' guidelines when prescribing antipsychotics to children and adolescents only about half the time, with failure to monitor cholesterol and blood sugar levels their main misstep."

## Advanced Monitoring

Several aspects of SGA monitoring are subtle, complex, or both, thus requiring additional training and skills. In monitoring for involuntary movements, particularly dyskinesias or akathisia, can be particularly challenging. Monitoring for any adverse effect during switching of SGAs can also be challenging.

### *Involuntary Movements*

The recommended method for assessing severity of abnormal involuntary movements[3] is to use a structured instrument, such as the Abnormal Involuntary Movements Scale (AIMS).[4] (See Appendix A.) It is important to obtain a baseline AIMS score before starting an SGA. Training in administration and scoring of the AIMS is recommended.[5]

**Table 6.5. Monitoring Protocol for [Adult] Patients on SGAs[a]**

| | Baseline | 4 weeks | 8 weeks | 12 weeks | Quarterly | Annually | Every 5 years |
|---|---|---|---|---|---|---|---|
| Personal/family history | X | | | | | X | |
| Weight (BMI) | X | X | X | X | X | | |
| Waist circumference | X | | | | | X | |
| Blood pressure | X | | | X | | X | |
| Fasting plasma glucose | X | | | X | | X | |
| Fasting lipid profile | X | | | X | | | X[b] |

Abbreviations: BMI, body mass index; SGA, second-generation antipsychotic.

[a] More frequent assessments may be warranted based on clinical status.

[b] Most proposed guidelines for children suggest annual monitoring of lipids, rather than every 5 years.

Adapted from American Diabetes Association, American Psychiatric Association, American Association of Clinical Endocrinologists, and North American Association for the Study of Obesity. Consensus Development Conference on Antipsychotic Drugs and Obesity and Diabetes. *Diabetes Care.* 2004;27(2):596–601. Copyright © 2004 American Diabetes Association.

Akathisia involves characteristic restless movements of the limbs, subjective awareness of restlessness, or both. Especially when mild, akathisia can be difficult to differentiate from fidgety movements. For eliciting subjective awareness, prompts such as "feeling like you have ants in your pants" or "feeling like you just swallowed some jumping beans" can be helpful. The Barnes Akathisia Rating Scale (BARS)[6] is the most commonly used structured instrument for rating severity of akathisia (see Appendix A for more information on BARS).

## Switching Second-Generation Antipsychotics

Switching SGAs in children and adolescents can be challenging and difficult, even in the hands of experienced specialists. Staggered switching is recommended to minimize symptomatic relapse. Because core psychiatric symptoms and adverse effects may emerge or increase during crossover of SGAs, monitoring requires extra vigilance. When possible, involving a child and adolescent psychiatrist or other experienced expert in switching SGAs is recommended.

## Comparing Second-Generation Antipsychotics

The following comments regarding differences between various Group 2 SGAs is offered as a general guide. It is not meant to create protocols for or restrict prescribing of any medication. An individualized decision regarding an individual medication for an individual patient is always the final responsibility of the individual prescriber.

No useful data compare efficacy of the 5 Group 2 SGAs in youth. Paliperidone is the active metabolite of risperidone and appears similar to risperidone in efficacy and adverse effect profile. Perhaps the major difference is that risperidone has been in use longer (since 1993) than paliperidone (since 2006) and is available as a generic formulation.

Generally, clinically meaningful differences between SGAs focus on adverse effects. Only a few relevant differences will be highlighted here. Olanzapine, in contrast with other Group 2 SGAs, is associated with more weight gain and metabolic adverse effects. Aripiprazole is associated with the least weight gain and less severe metabolic adverse effects. Among the 4, risperidone is most likely to increase prolactin levels and is more frequently associated with gynecomastia and amenorrhea (although there is not a consistent direct relationship between prolactin levels and these adverse effects). Quetiapine appears to be the most sedating. Detailed information regarding each Group 2 SGA is presented in Table 6.6.

**Table 6.6. Group 2 Medications: Second-Generation Antipsychotics**

| Medication | Warnings, Precautions, and Adverse Effects | Comments |
|---|---|---|
| **Risperidone**<br>*Indications in children and adolescents: Schizo-*phrenia (13–17 years), acute manic or mixed episodes (10–17 years), "irritability" associated with autism spectrum disorder (5–16 years)<br><br>*Uses:* Schizophrenia spectrum disorder, bipolar spectrum disorder, "irritability" in autism; also, among many off-label uses, acute aggression, chronic irritability, tics, and other disorders not responsive to other medications<br><br>*Monitoring:* See Tables 6.9 and 6.10 and Adverse Effects and Monitoring section of text. | *Boxed warnings:* Suicidality with antidepressant drugs<br><br>*Warnings and precautions:* Increased risk of suicidality in children, adolescents, and young adults with major depressive disorder, neuroleptic malignant syndrome, tardive dyskinesia, hyperglycemia and diabetes mellitus, dyslipidemia, weight gain, orthostatic hypotension, leukopenia, neutropenia, agranulocytosis, seizures and convulsions, potential for cognitive and motor impairment, suicide<br><br>*Adverse effects:* In children and adolescent clinical trials (incidence ≥5% and twice the placebo rate): somnolence, extrapyramidal disorder, fatigue, nausea, akathisia, blurred vision, salivary hypersecretion, dizziness, tremor, sedation, fatigue, increased appetite, drooling, vomiting, pyrexia, decreased appetite, lethargy | Risperidone was the first SGA (other than Clozaril, which is rarely used in children) approved by the FDA (in 1993) for marketing in the United States. It is generally effective and safe for short-term use, but there are concerns about adverse effects of long-term use, such as obesity, diabetes, metabolic syndrome, and tardive dyskinesia. It can increase prolactin levels and is associated with gynecomastia and amenorrhea. |
| **Aripiprazole**<br>*Indications in children and adolescents:* Schizophrenia (13–17 years), manic or mixed episodes (10–17 years), "irritability" associated with autism spectrum disorder (6–17 years)<br><br>*Uses:* Same as risperidone<br><br>*Monitoring:* Same as risperidone | Same as risperidone | Marketed since 2002, aripiprazole has a somewhat different mechanism of action than other SGAs. It is associated with less weight gain, except ziprasidone. It also lowers prolactin levels. |
| **Quetiapine**<br>*Indications in children and adolescents:* Schizophrenia (13–17 years), manic episodes associated with bipolar I disorder (10–17 years)<br><br>*Uses:* Same as risperidone<br><br>*Monitoring:* Same as risperidone | Same as risperidone | Marketed since 1997, quetiapine is associated with more somnolence than other SGAs. |

*continued on next page*

**Table 6.6 (continued)**

| Medication | Warnings, Precautions, and Adverse Effects | Comments |
|---|---|---|
| **Olanzapine**<br>*Indications in children and adolescents:* Schizophrenia (13–17 years), manic or mixed episodes of bipolar I disorder (13–17 years)<br>*Uses:* Same as risperidone<br>*Monitoring:* Same as risperidone | *Boxed warnings:* None specifically applicable for pediatrics<br><br>*Warnings and precautions:* Suicide, neuroleptic malignant syndrome, hyperglycemia, hyperlipidemia, tardive dyskinesia, orthostatic hypotension, leukopenia, neutropenia and agranulocytosis, seizures, potential for cognitive and motor impairment, hyperprolactinemia<br><br>*Adverse effects:* In adolescent clinical trials (incidence ≥5% and at least twice that for placebo): somnolence, dizziness, fatigue, increased appetite, nausea, vomiting, dry mouth, tachycardia, weight gain | Marketed since 1996, olanzapine is associated with more weight gain and related metabolic side effects in adolescents than other SGAs.[7,8] |
| **Paliperidone**<br>*Indications in children and adolescents:* Schizophrenia (12–17 years)<br>*Uses:* Same as risperidone<br>*Monitoring:* Same as risperidone | *Boxed warnings:* None specifically applicable for pediatrics<br><br>*Warnings and precautions:* Neuroleptic malignant syndrome, QT prolongation, tardive dyskinesia, hyperglycemia and diabetes mellitus, hyperglycemia, dyslipidemia, weight gain, hyperprolactinemia, gastrointestinal narrowing, orthostatic hypotension and syncope, leukopenia, neutropenia, agranulocytosis, potential for cognitive and motor impairment, seizures, suicide<br><br>*Adverse events:* The most common adverse reactions in adolescent clinical trials (≥5%) were somnolence, akathisia, tremor, dystonia, cogwheel rigidity, anxiety, weight gain, tachycardia | Because paliperidone is the major active metabolite of risperidone, it is very similar to risperidone in all respects. |

Abbreviation: FDA, Food and Drug Administration; SGA, second-generation antipsychotic.

# The Mood Stabilizer Lithium

Mood stabilizers (excluding antipsychotics) have mood-stabilizing effects and are used to treat mania, depression, irritability, and problematic mood swings or instability in bipolar disorder, as well as other mood disorders. There are 2 groups of mood stabilizers.

- Traditional (lithium, valproic acid [divalproex sodium], and carbamazepine)
- Newer anticonvulsants (eg, lamotrigine)

Use of mood stabilizers (excluding SGAs) in youth appears to be decreasing. This may be due to one or more factors.

- Available efficacy data for mania in bipolar disorder generally shows insignificant or minimal separation from placebo.
- Regular monitoring of plasma levels is usually required.
- The adverse effect burden is substantial.

Lithium is the mood stabilizer included in Group 2. Lithium has an FDA indication for mania in bipolar disorder down to age 12, and available data for lithium suggest efficacy for acute mania in bipolar disorder.[9,10] Detailed information regarding lithium is presented in Table 6.7.

Common adverse effects associated with lithium are presented in Box 6.6. Gastrointestinal problems (nausea, vomiting, diarrhea) and increased urination are common and are generally responsive to dose reduction.

Lithium has a narrow therapeutic window, and, as noted in the FDA boxed warning, toxicity is closely related to serum levels and can occur at doses close to therapeutic dosages.

As shown in Table 6.8, monitoring of lithium includes a targeted history, targeted physical examination, vital signs, and blood sampling. There is no formal schedule for monitoring. Generally, frequent serum lithium level monitoring (approximately 12 hours after the last dose) during dose escalation (generally no more frequently than 5 days following the most recent change in dose so that a steady state level has been reached) is optimal, until a stable and therapeutic blood level is reached. During maintenance treatment, monitoring, including serum blood levels, is generally recommended every 3 months. The target therapeutic level for bipolar disorder is generally in the 0.8 to 1.2 mEq/L. Therefore, safe prescribing of lithium necessitates an intensive monitoring regimen to ensure patient safety.

**Table 6.7. Group 2 Medications: Mood Stabilizer**

| Medication | Warnings, Precautions, and Adverse Effects | Comments |
|---|---|---|
| **Lithium**<br>*Class:* Element of the alkali-metal group (salt)<br><br>*Indications in children and adolescents:* Mania in bipolar disorder (age >12 years)<br><br>*Uses:* Acute mania and maintenance therapy in bipolar disorder, mood stabilization<br><br>*Monitoring:* Pregnancy testing; ECG; laboratory tests: serum lithium levels, CBC, electrolyte level, thyroid functions, and renal function | *Boxed warnings:* Toxicity closely related to serum levels; can occur close to therapeutic dose levels<br><br>*Warnings:* Very high risk of toxicity, including significant cardiovascular or renal disease, severe debilitation, dehydration, sodium depletion. Taking diuretics or ACE inhibitors. Chronic use may lower renal-concentrating ability and can present as nephrogenic diabetes insipidus, with polyuria or polydipsia. Encephalopathic syndrome (ie, weakness, lethargy, fever, tremulousness and confusion, leukocytosis, extrapyramidal symptoms, elevated serum enzyme level, BUN, and fasting blood glucose may occur with lithium and a neuroleptic, often haloperidol.<br><br>*Precautions:* Hypothyroidism, impaired mental or physical abilities, any concomitant medications (ie, diuretics, ACE inhibitors, carbamazepine, fluoxetine)<br><br>*Adverse effects:*<br>Mild: <1.5 mEq/L<br>Mild to moderate: 1.5–2.5 mEq/L<br>Moderate to severe: ≥2.0 mEq/L<br><2.0 mEq/L: Early signs of toxicity–diarrhea, vomiting, drowsiness, muscular weakness, and lack of coordination; at higher levels, giddiness, ataxia, blurred vision, tinnitus, large output of dilute urine<br>>3.0 mEq/L: Complex clinically, with multiple organs and organ systems | Introduced in the United States in the early 1960s, it was the original mood stabilizer. Clear, documented evidence of effectiveness for acute and maintenance treatment for mania and bipolar disorder in adults. No well-powered, placebo-controlled study for mania in children and adolescents, in large part, because of ethical and practical difficulties associated with conducting placebo-controlled studies. Evidence is mixed from several smaller studies.[9,10] Indication for 12- to 17-year-olds is not based on rigorous safety and efficacy data. Unpopular with children and adolescents because of common adverse effects and need for repeated venipunctures for serum level monitoring. |

Abbreviations: ACE, angiotensin-converting enzyme; BUN, blood urea nitrogen; CBC, complete blood count; ECG, electrocardiogram.

**Box 6.6. Common Adverse Effects and Laboratory Changes Associated With Lithium**

| |
|---|
| **Weight Gain** |
| **Gastrointestinal**<br>Nausea, vomiting, diarrhea |
| **Central Nervous System**<br>Slowing, tremor, ataxia |
| **Dermatologic**<br>Acne, rash |
| **Endocrine**<br>Thyroid dysfunction |
| **Renal**<br>Increased urination, renal function changes |

**Table 6.8. Lithium Monitoring**

| |
|---|
| **History** focused on adverse effects (baseline and at each follow-up visit) |
| **Physical Examination** focused on adverse effects, central nervous system, thyroid (baseline and at each follow-up visit) |
| **Vital Signs** (baseline, 3 months, 6 months, then annually)<br>Height, weight, blood pressure, and pulse |

**Laboratory Tests**

| System | Measure | Schedule |
|---|---|---|
| Lithium | 12-hour serum trough level (≥5 days' stable dose) | Baseline, during dose escalation, then every 3 months |
| General health | CBC | Baseline, then annually |
| Thyroid | TSH test | Baseline, 6 months, 12 months, then annually |
| Renal | Electrolyte, BUN, creatinine levels | Baseline, 3 months, 6 months, 12 months, then annually |
| Reproductive | HCG test | Baseline, then as indicated |
| Cardiac | ECG | Baseline, 3 months, 12 months, then annually |

Abbreviations: BUN, blood urea nitrogen; CBC, complete blood count; ECG, electrocardiogram; HCG, human chorionic gonadotropin; THS, thyroid-stimulating hormone.

Adapted from Ng F, Mammen OK, Wilting I, et al. The International Society for Bipolar Disorders (ISBD) consensus guidelines for the safety monitoring of bipolar disorder treatments. *Bipolar Disord.* 2009;11(6): 559–595 and Thomas T, Stansifer L, Findling RL. Psychopharmacology of pediatric bipolar disorders in children and adolescents. *Pediatr Clin North Am.* 2011; 58(1):173–187.

# Summary

Unifying characteristics of Group 2 medications are their association with substantial and potentially long-term adverse effects and their extensive monitoring protocols. Pediatric PCCs are ideally trained and skilled to provide this monitoring because they can integrate knowledge about the child's full health history to assess vulnerability to long-term adverse effects. For example, the pediatric PCC will likely know if the child has a family history of diabetes and if body mass index percentile of child has changed over time. Also, the pediatric PCC is likely to be comfortable with, and equipped to carry out, extensive monitoring protocols associated with Group 2 medications.

# References

1.  Leucht S, Samara M, Heres S, Patel MX, Woods SW, Davis JM. Dose equivalents for second-generation antipsychotics: the minimum effective dose method. *Schizophr Bull.* 2014;40(2):314–326
2.  Rettew DC, Greenblatt J, Kamon J, et al. Antipsychotic medication prescribing in children enrolled in Medicaid. *Pediatrics.* 2015;135(4):658–665
3.  American Academy of Child and Adolescent Psychiatry. Practice parameter for the assessment and treatment of children and adolescents with schizophrenia. *J Am Acad Child Adolesc Psychiatry.* 2001;40(7 Suppl):4S–23S
4.  Lane RD, Glazer WM, Hansen TE, Berman WH, Kramer SI. Assessment of tardive dyskinesia using the Abnormal Involuntary Movement Scale. *J Nerv Ment Dis.* 1985;173(6):353–357
5.  Munetz MR, Benjamin S. How to examine patients using the Abnormal Involuntary Movement Scale. *Hosp Community Psychiatry.* 1988;39(11):1172–1177
6.  Barnes TR. A rating scale for drug-induced akathisia. *Br J Psychiatry.* 1989;154:672–676
7.  Correll CU, Manu P, Olshanskiy V, Napolitano B, Kane JM, Malhotra AK. Cardiometabolic risk of second-generation antipsychotic medications during first-time use in children and adolescents. *JAMA.* 2009;302(16):1765–1773
8.  Correll CU, Sheridan EM, DelBello MP. Antipsychotic and mood stabilizer efficacy and tolerability in pediatric and adult patients with bipolar I mania: a comparative analysis of acute, randomized, placebo-controlled trials. *Bipolar Disord.* 2010;12(2):116–141
9.  Geller B, Luby JL, Joshi P, et al. A randomized controlled trial of risperidone, lithium, or divalproex sodium for initial treatment of bipolar I disorder, manic or mixed phase, in children and adolescents. *Arch Gen Psychiatry.* 2012;69(5):515–528
10. Robb AS, McNamara N, Pavuluri MN, et al. New research poster presentation 4.47. Lithium in the acute treatment of a manic or mixed episode in pediatric bipolar I disorder: a randomized, double-blind, placebo-controlled study. Abstract from the Annual Meeting of the American Academy of Child and Adolescent Psychiatry; October 2014; San Diego, CA.

# CHAPTER 7

# Group 3 Medications

Group 3 includes medications not approved for youth by the US Food and Drug Administration (FDA), thus not included in Groups 1 or 2.

A few other medications (not included in Groups 1 and 2) have FDA indications for youth, but these are based on premodern data (if there are any data) and were "grandfathered in" by the FDA years ago. Although the FDA has removed most of these grandfathered indications, a few remain. The author has excluded these approvals from this conceptual framework because they were not subject to the same modern standards of evidence for safety and efficacy as medications included in Groups 1 and 2.

For Group 3, 10 medications were selected for emphasis because they are commonly used and pediatric primary care clinicians (pediatric PCCs) are likely to have patients for whom they have been prescribed. Table 7.1 summarizes available efficacy data and adverse effect profiles for these 10 medications. Adverse effect data is taken from package inserts and is based on data from adult studies, as there are no applicable data for children younger than 18 years that the FDA has provided.

Other Group 3 medications, which are less commonly prescribed, will not be discussed, but their adverse effect profiles can be accessed via electronic media (eg, Drugs@FDA, Epocrates, Micromedex).

## Other Antidepressants

Four antidepressants—bupropion, citalopram, venlafaxine, and mirtazapine—are commonly prescribed in children and adolescents. None have FDA indications for use in children or adolescents.

*Bupropion* has a chemical structure similar to phenylethylamine, which is a stimulant. It is marketed for depression in adults and is sometimes used to treat comorbid depression and attention-deficit/hyperactivity disorder (ADHD) in youth.

**Table 7.1. Group 3 Medications**

| Medication | Warnings, Precautions, and Adverse Effects | Comments |
|---|---|---|
| **Antidepressant** | | |
| **Bupropion**<br>*Class:* Atypical antidepressant; chemical structure like phenylethylamine, which is a stimulant<br>*Indications*<br>  Adults: MDD<br>  Children and adolescents: None<br>*Uses:* Depression<br>*Monitoring:* BP, heart rate, height, weight, suicidality | *Boxed warnings:* Suicidality<br>*Warnings and precautions:* Seizures, hepatotoxicity, agitation and insomnia, psychosis and confusion, weight gain or loss, allergic reactions, hypertension<br>*Adverse effects:* Agitation, dry mouth, insomnia, headache and migraine, nausea and vomiting, constipation, tremor | Because of its structural similarity to stimulants, bupropion is sometimes used to treat both depression and symptoms of ADHD. |
| **Citalopram**<br>*Class:* SSRI<br>*Indications*<br>  Adult: MDD<br>  Children and adolescents: None<br>*Uses:* MDD<br>*Monitoring:* Same as other SSRIs (See Group 1.) | *Boxed warnings:* Suicidality, ECG changes<br>*Warnings and precautions:* Similar to other SSRIs<br>*Adverse effects:* Similar to other SSRIs | Offers no benefit over escitalopram, which is the Group 1 therapeutically effective (S)-enantiomer of citalopram. Also, citalopram has a US FDA warning regarding maximum dose in adults because of the risk of QTc prolongation; relevant dosage maximum is not known in children and adolescents. Thus, the potential need to monitor with ECGs complicates treatment. |
| **Venlafaxine**<br>*Class:* NRI<br>*Indications*<br>  Adult: MDD<br>  Children and adolescents: None[1,2]<br>*Uses:* MDD<br>*Monitoring:* BP, heart rate, height, weight, suicidality | *Boxed warnings:* Suicidality<br>*Warnings and precautions:* Serotonin syndrome, sustained hypertension, mydriasis, discontinuation symptoms—especially anxiety and insomnia, decreased appetite and weight, height deceleration, activation of mania and hypomania, hyponatremia, seizures, increased risk of bleeding events, serum cholesterol level elevation, interstitial lung disease, eosinophilic pneumonia<br>*Adverse effects:* Asthenia, sweating, nausea, constipation, anorexia, vomiting, somnolence, dry mouth, dizziness, nervousness, anxiety, tremor, blurred vision | Venlafaxine was compared with an SSRI in children and adolescents with depression who had not responded to initial treatment.[3] The second SSRI and venlafaxine showed comparable efficacy; however, venlafaxine was associated with more adverse effects and discontinuations. |

**Mirtazapine**
*Class:* Tetracyclic
*Indications*
　Adult: MDD
　Children and adolescents: None
*Uses:* MDD
*Monitoring:* BMI, WBC count, lipid panel, transaminase level

*Boxed warnings:* Suicidality
*Warnings:* Activation of mania and hypomania, agranulocytosis, serotonin syndrome, angle-closure glaucoma
*Precautions:* Discontinuation symptoms, akathisia, hyponatremia, somnolence, dizziness, increased appetite and weight gain, cholesterol and triglyceride levels, transaminase level elevation, seizures
*Adverse effects:* Somnolence, increased appetite, weight gain, dizziness

Mirtazapine has both serotonergic and nor-adrenergic actions and is different from other antidepressants in its mechanism of action. It is generally more sedating and causes more weight gain than other antidepressants. Because of its sedating effect, it is sometimes used as a sleep aid.

## Second-Generation Antipsychotic

**Ziprasidone**
*Class:* SGA
*Indications*
　Adult: Schizophrenia, manic or mixed episodes associated with bipolar I disorder, adjunctive maintenance therapy of bipolar I disorder, agitation in schizophrenic patients (intramuscular injection)
　Children and Adolescents: None
*Uses:* Same as risperidone (See Group 2 SGAs.)
*Monitoring:* Same as risperidone, plus QTc on ECG

*Boxed warnings:* Increased mortality in elderly patients
*Warnings and precautions:* QT interval prolongation, neuroleptic malignant syndrome, tardive dyskinesia, hyperglycemia and diabetes mellitus, dyslipidemia, rash, orthostatic hypotension, leukopenia, neutropenia, agranulocytosis, seizures, potential for cognitive and motor impairment, suicide
*Adverse effects:* Most common adverse effects in clinical trials (incidence ≥5% and twice placebo): somnolence, respiratory tract infection, somnolence, extrapyramidal symptoms, dizziness, akathisia, abnormal vision, asthenia, vomiting, extrapyramidal symptoms, dizziness, akathisia, abnormal vision, asthenia, vomiting, headache, nausea

Marketed since 2001, ziprasidone is associated with less weight gain than other SGAs. Because of potential to prolong the QT interval, ECG monitoring is needed.

*continued on next page*

**Table 7.1 (continued)**

| Medication | Warnings, Precautions, and Adverse Effects | Comments |
|---|---|---|
| **Mood Stabilizer** | | |
| ***Valproic Acid***<br>*Class:* Anticonvulsant mood stabilizer<br>*Indications*<br>Adult: Therapy of complex partial seizures and simple and complex absence seizures<br>Children and adolescents: None psychiatric<br>*Uses:* Mood stabilizer<br>*Monitoring:* Pregnancy testing, serum levels, CBC, liver function tests | *Boxed warnings:* Hepatotoxicity—can be fatal, usually in first 6 months of use in children <2 years; teratogenic, including neural tube defects (eg, spina bifida, malformations, decreased IQ; pancreatitis—can be fatal, hemorrhagic cases<br>*Warnings and precautions:* Hepatotoxicity, birth defects and decreased IQ following in utero exposure, pancreatitis, suicidality, thrombocytopenia, multiorgan hypersensitivity reaction, hypothermia, hyperammonemia, hyperammonemic encephalopathy, multiorgan hypersensitivity reaction<br>*Adverse effects:* Most common adverse effects in clinical trials of mania (incidence ≥5%): abdominal pain, alopecia, amblyopia and blurred vision, amnesia, anorexia, asthenia, ataxia, bronchitis, constipation, depression, diarrhea, diplopia, dizziness, dyspepsia, dyspnea, ecchymosis, emotional lability, fever, flu syndrome, headache, increased appetite, infection, insomnia, nausea, nervousness, nystagmus, peripheral edema, pharyngitis, rhinitis, somnolence, abnormal thinking, thrombocytopenia, tinnitus, tremor, vomiting, weight gain, weight loss | Valproic acid for treatment of mania in adults is supported by substantial data. Supportive data are lacking in youth. An industry-funded, multisite RCT in youth with mania in bipolar disorder did not show efficacy of valproic acid versus placebo.[4] In a comparison of valproic acid, lithium and risperidone for bipolar disorder in youth,[5] valproic acid had the lowest response rates; they were comparable to those for placebo in the industry-funded study. |

## Anxiolytics

**Lorazepam**
*Class:* Benzodiazepine
*Indications*
  Adult: Acute anxiety
  Children and adolescents: None
*Uses:* Acute anxiety
*Monitoring:* Pregnancy testing

*Boxed warnings:* None
*Warnings:* Worsening or emergence of depression, suicidality, respiratory depression, interference with cognitive and motor performance, physical and psychologic dependence, risk of use in pregnancy, withdrawal symptoms
*Precautions:* Paradoxical reactions (ie, behavioral disinhibition), should not be used with alcohol
*Adverse effects:* In a sample of about 3,500 adult patients treated for anxiety, the most frequent adverse effect was sedation (15.9%), followed by dizziness (6.9%), weakness (4.2%), and unsteadiness (3.4%).

Lorazepam is a short-acting benzodiazepine with a duration of effect of about 4–8 hours. Primarily because of the possibility of physical and psychological dependence with prolonged use of benzodiazepines, lorazepam is generally recommended only for short-term use (days to a few weeks) for treatment of acute and severe anxiety following a trauma, preceding a medical procedure, or while waiting for an SSRI or other anxiolytic to become effective.

**Clonazepam**
*Class:* Benzodiazepine
*Indications*
  Adult: Panic disorder
  Children and adolescents: None
*Uses:* Acute anxiety
*Monitoring:* Pregnancy testing

*Boxed warnings:* None
*Warnings:* Interference with cognitive and motor performance, suicidality, physical and psychologic dependence, risk of use in pregnancy, withdrawal symptoms
*Precautions:* Worsening of seizures, hypersalivation, should not be used with alcohol
*Adverse effects:* Somnolence, coordination abnormal, ataxia, depression

Clonazepam is similar to lorazepam, except for its longer half-life and once-daily dosing.

*continued on next page*

**Table 7.1** *(continued)*

| Medication | Warnings, Precautions, and Adverse Effects | Comments |
|---|---|---|
| **Sleep Aids** | | |
| **Trazodone**<br>*Class:* Serotonergic potentiator with unclear specific mechanism of action<br>*Indications*<br>Adult: MDD<br>Children and adolescents: None<br>*Uses:* Insomnia<br>*Monitoring:* Pregnancy testing | *Boxed warnings:* Suicidality<br>*Warnings and precautions:* Serotonin syndrome, angle closure glaucoma, activation of mania and hypomania, QT prolongation, orthostatic hypotension and syncope, abnormal bleeding, interaction with MAOIs, priapism, hyponatremia, potential for cognitive and motor impairment, discontinuation syndrome<br>*Adverse effects:* Somnolence and sedation, dizziness, constipation, blurred vision | Trazodone is sometimes used as a sleep aid in low doses, generally 25 or 50 mg. Because of reports of priapism, its use in adolescent boys is limited. |

Abbreviations: ADHD, attention-deficit/hyperactivity disorder; BMI, body mass index; BP, blood pressure; ECG, electrocardiogram; FDA, Food and Drug Administration; MAOI, monoamine oxidase inhibitor; MDD, major depressive disorder; NRI, norepinephrine reuptake inhibitor; RCT, randomized controlled trial; SSRI, selective serotonin reuptake inhibitor; WBC, white blood cell.

Although *citalopram*, a selective serotonin reuptake inhibitor (SSRI), is sometimes used for depression, anxiety, or both in youth, it offers no benefit over escitalopram, a Group 1 medication that is the therapeutically effective (*S*)-enantiomer of citalopram. Citalopram has an FDA warning regarding maximum dose in adults because of the risk of QTc prolongation; however, a relevant dosage maximum is not known in children and adolescents. Thus, the need to monitor with electrocardiograms complicates treatment in pediatric patients.

*Venlafaxine* is a norepinephrine reuptake inhibitor that "behaves" like an SSRI at lower doses. It is used for anxiety, depression, or both in youth.[1,2] In children and adolescents, venlafaxine is associated with more adverse effects than SSRIs.[3] Industry-sponsored efficacy studies for depression and anxiety in youth, although almost reaching statistical significance, have not demonstrated clear efficacy.[1,2]

*Mirtazapine* has a tetracyclic chemical structure that distinguishes it from other antidepressants. It is marketed for depression in adults. Mirtazapine is associated with more sedation and weight gain than other antidepressants.

## Other Antipsychotics

*Ziprasidone* is a second-generation antipsychotic (marked since 2001) that is approved in adults for psychosis in schizophrenia and mania in bipolar disorder. Ziprasidone has the advantage of generally being associated with less weight gain and fewer metabolic adverse effects than other second-generation antipsychotics. However, it is associated with prolongation of QTc and has not been approved by the FDA for children or adolescents.

## Other Mood Stabilizers

*Divalproex* sodium, an anticonvulsant, is commonly prescribed to youth as a mood stabilizer. Unfortunately, efficacy data for divalproex sodium for mania in bipolar disorder suggest no difference from placebo[4] and less efficacy than comparators.[6] Adverse effect burden is considerable, and monitoring requires regular venipunctures.

# Anxiolytics

Two benzodiazepine anxiolytics—*lorazepam* (short acting) and clonaze-pam (long acting)—are commonly prescribed in children and adolescents. Because dependence may develop with long-term benzodiazepine treatment, they are recommended for short-term use *only*.

Benzodiazepines may be used prior to painful or stressful medical proce-dures. They can be used for short-term treatment of anxiety and distress following an acute traumatic incident or while waiting for an SSRI to have an effect. Also, benzodiazepines are used as an adjunctive treatment of schizophrenia.

Benzodiazepines are generally well tolerated. Sedation is the most common concerning adverse effect. Daytime drowsiness can be dangerous when oper-ating a motor vehicle or machinery. In children, benzodiazepines, especially at relatively low doses, can cause generalized verbal and physical disinhibition, which appears to be most common in children with intellectual and neuro-developmental disorders. Other concerning adverse effects are unlikely if benzodiazepines are used short-term and at appropriately low doses.

# Sleep Aids

Insomnia is a common concern in youth with ADHD, anxiety, depression, and other disorders. In general, treatment of the primary psychiatric disor-der(s), plus counseling, behavioral approaches, or both to improving sleep hygiene, will relieve insomnia. If not, further evaluation is recommended.

Although research data are lacking, various medications are used to treat in-somnia in children and adolescents, especially those with ADHD or autism spectrum disorder associated with sleep problems. Two potential sleep aids, which are among the most commonly used in youth, are included here.

*Trazodone* is an antidepressant approved for treatment of major depressive disorder in adults. It is sometimes used in low doses to treat insomnia in adolescents (and adults). Trazodone's mechanism of action is not well under-stood; its major effect is thought to be on the serotonergic system. Trazo-done's adverse effects profile is similar to the SSRIs, but it is also associated with priapism, which may limit its use in male adolescents.

*Melatonin* is a hormone produced in the pineal gland and is available over the counter (OTC) but not by prescription (and therefore is not included in Table 7.1). This is a problem because the FDA does not monitor quality control of such OTC preparations; thus, the actual dose in an OTC melatonin preparation may not be the same as the dose on the label. Melatonin appears to be effective in reducing time to sleep onset in adults (and, based on considerably less data, in children) with initial insomnia. This effect appears to last for days to weeks but not long-term. Thus, melatonin is not recommended for long-term use. It may be helpful for short-term alleviation of initial insomnia, which is relatively common following severe trauma, during an episode of depression, or following travel that crosses multiple time zones. Melatonin's primary adverse effect is sedation.

## Future Considerations

The medications included in Groups 1, 2, and 3 were based on data available as of March 5, 2015. Medications included in Groups 1 and 2 will change as new medications obtain FDA approval for children and adolescents.

Medications included in Group 3 will change as medications without FDA approval in youth become more commonly used or if a medication included in Group 3 gains FDA approval and moves to Groups 1 or 2. A potential example is the antipsychotic ziprasidone, which, if it gained FDA approval in youth, would move from Group 3 to Group 2.

A potential example of a medication that could move onto the Group 3 list, if it becomes commonly used in children or adolescents, is ramelteon. Ramelteon is a recently FDA-approved sleep aid (for adults only) that is the first in a new class of sleep aids that are melatonin (MT) receptor agonists with high affinity for MT1 and MT2 receptors. At this time, though, ramelteon is too new to allow an informed assessment of its appropriateness for children and adolescents.

## References

1.  Brent D, Emslie G, Clarke G, et al. Switching to another SSRI or to venlafaxine with or without cognitive behavioral therapy for adolescents with SSRI-resistant depression: the TORDIA randomized controlled trial. *JAMA.* 2008;299(8):901–913

2. Rynn MA, Riddle MA, Yeung PP, Kunz NR. Efficacy and safety of extended-release venlafaxine in the treatment of generalized anxiety disorder in children and adolescents: two placebo-controlled trials. *Am J Psychiatry.* 2007;164(2):290–300

3. Emslie GJ, Findling RL, Yeung PP, Kunz NR, Li Y. Venlafaxine ER for the treatment of pediatric subjects with depression: results of two placebo-controlled trials. *J Am Acad Child Adolesc Psychiatry.* 2007;46(4):479–488

4. Wagner KD, Redden L, Kowatch RA, et al. A double-blind, randomized, placebo-controlled trial of divalproex extended-release in the treatment of bipolar disorder in children and adolescents. *J Am Acad Child Adolesc Psychiatry.* 2009;48(5):519–532

5. Geller B, Luby JL, Joshi P, et al. A randomized controlled trial of risperidone, lithium, or divalproex sodium for initial treatment of bipolar I disorder, manic or mixed phase, in children and adolescents. *Arch Gen Psychiatry.* 2012;69(5):515–528

6. American Diabetes Association, American Psychiatric Association, American Association of Clinical Endocrinologists, North American Association for the Study of Obesity. Consensus development conference on antipsychotic drugs and obesity and diabetes. *Diabetes Care.* 2004;27(2):596–601

# Part 5—Advanced Topics

# CHAPTER 8

# What to Do When Treatment Is Not Successful

## The Limits of Evidence-Based Treatments and Protocols

This chapter addresses the question "What should you do when treatment is not successful?"

While evidence-based treatments recommended in this book can be expected to substantially reduce symptoms and improve function in most children and adolescents, nonresponse or partial response to treatment is not unusual. Placebo-controlled studies indicate that about 10% to 40% of patients do not respond to an initial intervention, depending on diagnosis and treatment. (Treatment that combines medication and evidence-based therapy leads to higher response rates in attention-deficit/hyperactivity disorder [ADHD], anxiety, and depression. Thus, whenever possible, it is important to recommend both medication and evidence-based therapy.)

An optimal time to reassess treatment is after a patient has received adequate dose and duration of medication, as well as (when applicable) adequate duration of psychotherapy and pragmatic support, yet is still unimproved or only partially improved.

## Reassess Diagnoses

The diagnostic approaches described in Chapter 2 should result in correct diagnoses for most patients. However, complex psychosocial presentations, multiple potential diagnoses, or both can complicate the assessment process. In addition, diagnosis often relies heavily upon parent and child report, which can be affected by differing perspectives of symptom severity.

## Incomplete or Inaccurate Reports

Examples of problems of incomplete or inaccurate reporting that can make correct diagnosis difficult include

- Minimization of symptoms by the patient or family because of concerns about stigma
- Misinterpreting normal behavior as symptomatic of a problem
- Fear of revealing symptoms for various reasons (eg, physical, psychological, or sexual abuse)
- Reluctance to reveal symptoms because of desire to be or appear "normal"
- Differing reports among various family members and the patient

Rating scales completed by both parents and teachers can be helpful in clarifying symptom type and severity. When considering whether behavior is normal, it may be helpful to remember that in one study, 13% of parents of school-aged children and 10% of parents of preschool-aged children with normal functioning reported concerns about their child's behavior.[1,2]

Inconsistencies between clinical evaluation and rating-scale data may also indicate that a teacher's expectation may not be consistent with the child's skill level. Having the rating scales completed by multiple teachers who see the child throughout the school day is often beneficial to identify which problems have a global effect on academic functioning.

Many teens are more comfortable reporting symptoms on paper or electronic forms than in individual or family interviews.

Rating scales can also help begin an open conversation about the child's strengths and challenges, which is especially important when differences between various reporting sources are present.

## Phenomenological or Nosologic Issues

Examples of phenomenological or nosologic issues that may make diagnostic clarity difficult include

- Impaired concentration may be a symptom of anxiety or depression, or secondary to trauma, rather than ADHD.
- Feelings associated with anxiety (eg, frustration, defeat) may be accompanied by more active symptoms, such as anger, aggression, and oppositional behavior, that "mask" anxiety symptoms.
- Demoralization (ie, loss of hope, confidence, courage) may be mistaken for depression or "defiance."

## ADHD

As a reminder, when the diagnosis of ADHD is in question, the most important data for diagnosing it in a child reflect caregivers' and teachers' observations that can be recorded and organized using structured rating scales. Some children with ADHD will exhibit hyperactivity, impulsivity, distractibility, or a combination of those in the examination room; however, many will not. Obtaining symptom information from informants over at least a week and during various times of day strengthens validity of the diagnosis, as symptom severity waxes and wanes over short periods.

## Anxiety Disorders

As a reminder, the core symptoms of anxiety disorders are

- Fears or phobias
- Worries
- Somatic concerns

A common response to these symptoms is avoidance of situations that generate fear or worry. Children with anxiety can present to the pediatric primary care clinician (pediatric PCC) in various ways. Children may share their worries, fears, or somatic concerns with their caregivers, who will describe them during an office visit. In other cases, a caregiver may report that a child is excessively shy or is avoiding social or other situations (eg, coming close to dogs, being alone). Sometimes, however, children keep their fears or worries to themselves and do not share them with others. Thus, a general inquiry regarding concerns, worries, and sources of discomfort may elicit previously unidentified anxiety. Anxiety and depression also frequently co-occur, with one set of symptoms and related behaviors exacerbating the other. When 1 of the 2 conditions is suspected, it is necessary to ask about the other as well.

## Depression

Differential diagnosis of major depressive disorder (MDD) in youth can be challenging. Children who are demoralized by various family, social, medical, peer, academic, or other problems can exhibit many of the symptoms of MDD. Demoralized children often have mood and cognitive symptoms identical to those in children with MDD, but neurovegetative symptoms are less likely to be present. Grief can also mimic MDD. The prominent affect in a grieving child is a feeling of emptiness or loss, in contrast with the child with MDD, whose prominent affect is depressed mood, the inability to anticipate happiness or pleasure, or both. Trauma- and stress-related disorders, such as adjustment disorder with depressed mood, may also mimic MDD. The essential distinguishing feature of adjustment disorder is an identifiable stressor that precedes mood symptoms.

## Reassess Non-diagnostic Issues and Concerns

In addition to reassessing diagnoses, it is important to reassess for relevant new information regarding

- History of present illness
- Past personal history
- Family history
- Family stressors and conflicts
- School stressors or problems
- Adverse childhood experiences
- Substance abuse
- Treatment adherence

Comments or questions that may be useful in reassessment include

- "Let's review and rethink some of the topics we discussed before."
- "Has anything happened since the initial evaluation that might help us understand why your child isn't getting better?"
- "Are you having any problems getting her to participate in therapy?"
- "Are there any problems with medication? Remembering to take it? Actually taking it?"
- "Are you having any problems with insurance or Medicaid when purchasing medication?"
- "Is there anything else we should be talking or thinking about?"

## Reconsider Psychotherapy(ies) or Therapist

If a patient is not improving and the treatment plan does not include evidence-based psychotherapy, adding therapy is recommended. Evidence-based psychotherapies are described and discussed in the Psychological Treatments section in Chapter 3. Generally, patients or families that have been reluctant to try psychotherapy will be more motivated if an initial treatment without evidence-based psychotherapy was unsuccessful.

If the patient is not improving and the treatment plan includes psychother-apy but not medication, it is recommended that reevaluation include the effectiveness of psychotherapy and whether the therapist is a good "fit" for this patient, before consideration of adding medication. In addition to re-evaluating with the patient and caregiver(s), discussing and reevaluating the treatment plan with the therapist can provide useful information about both the psychotherapy and the therapist's approach and fit.

If the patient is not improving and the treatment plan includes medication and therapy, both need to be reevaluated. Changing only one or the other is recommended. Changing medication and therapy simultaneously makes it difficult to determine which treatment is having what effect.

# Reconsider Medication

## When Medication Is Ineffective

If the first medication is not effective, there is some evidence to support switching to a second medication.

For ADHD, when the initial stimulant fails, available evidence supports switching from an amphetamine to a methylphenidate preparation or vice versa. About 70% of children with ADHD respond to either methylphenidate or amphetamine. Evidence suggests that almost all children with ADHD respond to the other type or class of stimulant if the first is ineffective.[3]

For depression, available evidence in adolescents suggests that if the first selective serotonin reuptake inhibitor (SSRI) is not effective, the optimal choice for a second medication is another SSRI.[4]

For anxiety, there are no data from rigorous studies regarding the best choice for a second medication, although extrapolation from the depression data[4] would support trying a second SSRI for anxiety.

No data support decisions about switching or adding medication if the first 2 medications (prescribed sequentially) have failed for ADHD, anxiety, or depression. Treatment algorithms have been published for various disor-ders,[5-7] but, beyond the second medication, they are based on expert opin-ion, not rigorous clinical research data. Thus, if 2 sequential medication trials have failed to yield a positive therapeutic response and adherence is consistent, consideration of consultation with a specialist or expert is recommended.

## When the First Medication Is Partially Effective

If the first medication is partially effective, addition of a second or "augmenting" medication may be indicated. The only available data supporting safe and effective combined medication treatment in youth are for guanfacine with methylphenidate for ADHD.[8,9] No such studies are available for youth with anxiety or depression.

## When Adverse Effects Lead to Discontinuation of a Medication

If the first medication needs to be stopped because of adverse effects, deciding which medication to recommend next may be more complicated.

For ADHD, trying the other type or class of stimulant, as described previously, is a viable option. Bypassing a second type or class of stimulant and recommending guanfacine or clonidine may be considered if, for example, the patient or caregiver(s) objects to a second stimulant.

For anxiety or depression, switching to another SSRI, as described previously, is generally recommended. However, especially if the patient or caregiver(s) objects, trying another class of antidepressant may be the next best option. See When to Consider Group 3 Medications Without FDA Approval for Use in Youth section later in this chapter for a discussion of such Group 3 medications.

# When to Consider Group 2 Antipsychotics or Lithium

As described in Chapter 6, several antipsychotics have FDA approval for short-term treatment of youth with psychosis in schizophrenia, mania in bipolar disorder, and "irritability" in autism spectrum disorder. Generally, they are prescribed by specialists with experience in treating these relatively uncommon disorders.

When a pediatric PCC is unable to obtain an appropriate consultation with, or referral to, a specialist, there may be circumstances when it is necessary for the pediatric PCC to prescribe an antipsychotic. In these circumstances, the National Network of Child Psychiatry Access Programs, a group of support programs in more than one-half of US states that provide consultations, may be helpful in providing relatively quick consultation and information about available resources (www.nncpap.org/existing-programs). They will usually provide these consultations by phone and at no charge. Specific information regarding antipsychotics with FDA approval for use in youth is available in Chapter 7.

Lithium is FDA approved for short-term treatment of mania in bipolar disorder in adolescents. Everything above about antipsychotics also applies to lithium, except for its singular indication.

Primary care monitoring of Group 2 medications ideally requires close collaboration between the PCC and a mental health specialist, much like the collaboration that takes place between the PCC and medical subspecialists, such as pulmonologists and cardiologists. Significant barriers to collaboration between PCCs and mental health specialists exist, including the misperception that the HIPAA (Health Information Portability and Accountability Act) prevents them from exchanging information without explicit patient consent. Although HIPAA allows exchange of information without the patient's consent between clinicians who are treating a common patient (except psychotherapy notes per se and certain information regarding substance abuse treatment services), PCCs are encouraged to obtain signed release of information forms so that exchange of mental health–related information between the PCC and specialty provider can be expedited. When possible, communication within an electronic health record is highly desirable, giving both PCC and specialist access to all relevant clinical information in real time. Developing relationships between a primary care office staff member and a staff member in the mental health specialist's office can also improve collaboration. The American Academy of Pediatrics *Addressing Mental Health Concerns in Primary Care: A Clinician's Toolkit* provides sample letters that can be used by PCCs to introduce their practice to mental health professionals in their community, obtain information from mental health professionals about services that they provide, and exchange feedback about their patient's progress.

Antipsychotics are used to treat youth with dysregulated (ie, erratic, rapidly changing) behavior or aggression more frequently than they are used to treat youth with disorders for which antipsychotics are indicated. Generally, a child or adolescent who needs an antipsychotic for dysregulated behavior and aggression also needs the resources of the mental and behavioral health system of care. Thus, it is recommended that, whenever possible, this off-label prescribing be done by specialists embedded in the mental and behavioral system of care and experienced in treating these often complex problems.

# When to Consider Group 3 Medications Without FDA Approval for Use in Youth

As described in Chapter 7, Group 3 medications are not FDA approved for use in youth with psychiatric disorders. Generally, they are prescribed by specialists for disorders other than ADHD, anxiety, and depression. When a pediatric PCC is unable to obtain an appropriate consultation with, or referral to, a specialist, there may be circumstances when it is necessary to prescribe a Group 3 medication. In these circumstances, as above, consultation with a child psychiatrist by phone or telemedicine link should be considered.

Information regarding 10 of the more commonly prescribed Group 3 medications is available in Chapter 7.

# When to Consider Drug Levels or Genetic Testing

## When Is a Drug Level Test Indicated?

Most children and adolescents' psychotropic medication can be effectively and safely managed without obtaining drug levels.

Although relatively rare, the most common indications for considering drug level testing are

- Inadequate response at maximum recommended total daily dose
- Worrisome adverse effects that persist at therapeutic doses
- Suspected non-adherence

Some psychotropic medications (eg, fluoxetine, risperidone) have active metabolites that are usually included in a "drug level" obtained from a reputable laboratory. Although there is no established therapeutic blood level for most psychotropic medications, levels that are undetectable, low, or high can be helpful in guiding treatment.

An "undetectable" drug (and, when applicable, active metabolite) level usually indicates non-adherence. A low drug level may indicate inconsistent adherence. Specific interventions to improve adherence,[10-14] referral to a specialist, or both may be useful. Continuing to increase dose in these situations is not recommended.

A low drug level may also indicate that the patient is an ultrarapid or extensive metabolizer of the drug. Increasing the dose above the recommended total daily maximum may be necessary to achieve a therapeutic response. Consistent and systematic monitoring for clinical response and adverse effects (or referral to a specialist) is obviously important in such situations.

A very high drug (and, when applicable, active metabolite) level in a patient on a total daily dose in the recommended dosing range may indicate that the patient is a poor metabolizer of the drug. Such patients frequently have concerning and persistent adverse effects. Lowering the total daily dose until adverse effects are manageable or nonexistent is the recommended intervention for these patients.

For medications with active metabolites that are reported by the laboratory, the ratio of the levels of the parent drug and active metabolite can be informative. Before making changes in dose based on ratios, consultation with an expert at the laboratory or an appropriate specialist is recommended.

## When Is Genotyping of CYP450 Isoenzymes Indicated?

Commercial vendors are increasingly promoting genotyping of CYP450 isoenzymes to assist in management of medication. In pediatric psychopharmacology, clinical genotyping of CYP450 isoenzymes is rarely indicated.

If dosage adjustment and use of drug levels does not result in an adequate outcome, it may be useful to establish the patient's metabolizer status (eg, poor, intermediate, extensive, ultrarapid) by genotyping the isoenzyme(s) (eg, CYP2D6 for fluoxetine; CYP3A4 for sertraline) involved primarily in metabolism of the particular medication.

# When to Consider Consultation or a Second Opinion

It is appropriate to seek consultation anytime a pediatric PCC has doubts or questions about an evaluation, treatment plan, or a patient's clinical status. Positing specific questions and concerns may improve quality of the consultative feedback. Pediatric PCCs are encouraged to establish relationships with mental health specialists in their community or with their regional medical center so that these issues can be addressed when concerns arise.

# When to Consider Referral for All or Part of the Patient's Ongoing Behavioral Health Care

Whenever a pediatric PCC feels that a patient's evaluation or treatment will require knowledge or skills beyond her or his repertoire, a referral to another clinician for part or all of the patient's mental and behavioral health care is recommended. Even when such a referral is for all mental and behavioral care, the pediatric PCC can play an important part in the patient's overall care, especially in monitoring medication adverse effects, encouraging the patient and family to continue the mental and behavioral health treatment, providing preventive services, and coordinating care of any comorbid medical conditions.

# References

1. Costello EJ, Edelbrock C, Costello AJ, Dulcan MK, Burns BJ, Brent D. Psychopathology in pediatric primary care: the new hidden morbidity. *Pediatrics.* 1988;82(3 Pt 2):415–424
2. Jellinek MS, Murphy JM, Little M, Pagano ME, Comer DM, Kelleher KJ. Use of the Pediatric Symptom Checklist to screen for psychosocial problems in pediatric primary care: a national feasibility study. *Arch Pediatr Adolesc Med.* 1999;153(3):254–260
3. Elia J, Borcherding BG, Rapoport JL, Keysor CS. Methylphenidate and dextroamphetamine treatments of hyperactivity: are there true nonresponders? *Psychiatry Res.* 1991;36(2):141–155
4. Brent D, Emslie G, Zelazny J, et al. Switching to another SSRI or to venlafaxine with or without cognitive behavioral therapy for adolescents with SSRI-resistant depression: the TORDIA randomized control trial. *JAMA.* 2008;299(8):901–913
5. Hughes CW, Emslie GJ, Crismon ML, et al. Texas Children's Medication Algorithm Project: update from Texas Consensus Conference Panel on Medication Treatment of Childhood Major Depressive Disorder. *J Am Acad Child Adolesc Psychiatry.* 2007;46(6):667–686
6. Pliszka SR, Crismon ML, Hughes CW, et al; Texas Consensus Conference Panel on Pharmacotherapy of Childhood Attention Deficit Hyperactivity Disorder. The Texas Children's Medication Algorithm Project: revision of the algorithm for pharmacotherapy of attention-deficit/hyperactivity disorder. *J Am Acad Child Adolesc Psychiatry.* 2006;45(6):642–657
7. American Academy of Pediatrics Steering Committee on Quality Improvement and Management, Subcommittee on Attention-Deficit/Hyperactivity Disorder. Implementing the key action statements: an algorithm and explanation for process of care for the evaluation, diagnosis, treatment, and monitoring of ADHD in children and adolescents. *Pediatrics.* 2011;128(5):SI1–SI21
8. Spencer TJ, Greenbaum M, Ginsberg LD, Murphy WR. Safety and effectiveness of coadministration of guanfacine extended release and psychostimulants in children and adolescents with attention-deficit/hyperactivity disorder. *J Child Adolesc Psychopharmacol.* 2009;19(5):501–510

9.  Wilens TE, Bukstein O, Brams M, et al. A controlled trial of extended-release guanfacine and psychostimulants for attention-deficit/hyperactivity disorder. *J Am Acad Child Adolesc Psychiatry.* 2012;51(1):74–85

10. Chong WW, Aslani P, Chen TF. Effectiveness of interventions to improve antidepressant medication adherence: a systematic review. *Int J Clin Pract.* 2011;65(9):954–975

11. Hamrin V, McGuinness TM. Motivational interviewing: a tool for increasing psychotropic medication adherence for youth. *J Psychosoc Nurs Ment Health Serv.* 2013;51(6): 15–18

12. McGuinness TM, Worley J. Promoting adherence to psychotropic medication for youth-part 1. *J Psychosoc Nurs Ment Health Serv.* 2010;48(10):19–22

13. McGuinness TM, Worley J. Promoting adherence to psychotropic medication for youth-part 2. *J Psychosoc Nurs Ment Health Serv.* 2010;48(10):22–26

14. Van Cleave J, Leslie LK. Approaching ADHD as a chronic condition: implications for long-term adherence. *J Psychosoc Nurs Ment Health Serv.* 2008;46(8):28–37

# Appendixes

# Assessment and Symptom Monitoring Tools

## Pediatric Symptom Checklist

The Pediatric Symptom Checklist (PSC) is a general screening tool for identifying emotional and behavioral concerns in youths aged 4 to 16 years. It is reproduced below and is available online at http://brightfutures.org /mentalhealth/pdf/professionals/ped_sympton_chklst.pdf. An abbreviated 17-item scale and a self-report version, for youths aged 11 and older, is also available.

BRIGHT FUTURES ☀ TOOL FOR PROFESSIONALS

I N S T R U C T I O N S    F O R    U S E

# Pediatric Symptom Checklist

The Pediatric Symptom Checklist is a psychosocial screen designed to facilitate the recognition of cognitive, emotional, and behavioral problems so that appropriate interventions can be initiated as early as possible. Included here are two versions, the parent-completed version (PSC) and the youth self-report (Y-PSC). The Y-PSC can be administered to adolescents ages 11 and up.

**INSTRUCTIONS FOR SCORING**

The PSC consists of 35 items that are rated as "Never," "Sometimes," or "Often" present and scored 0, 1, and 2, respectively. The total score is calculated by adding together the score for each of the 35 items. For children and adolescents ages 6 through 16, a cutoff score of 28 or higher indicates psychological impairment. For children ages 4 and 5, the PSC cutoff score is 24 or higher (Little et al., 1994; Pagano et al., 1996). The cutoff score for the Y-PSC is 30 or higher. Items that are left blank are simply ignored (i.e., score equals 0). If four or more items are left blank, the questionnaire is considered invalid.

**HOW TO INTERPRET THE PSC OR Y-PSC**

A positive score on the PSC or Y-PSC suggests the need for further evaluation by a qualified health (e.g., M.D., R.N.) or mental health (e.g., Ph.D., L.I.C.S.W.) professional. Both false positives and false negatives occur, and only an experienced health professional should interpret a positive PSC or Y-PSC score as anything other than a suggestion that further evaluation may be helpful. Data from past studies using the PSC and Y-PSC indicate that two out of three children and adolescents who screen positive on the PSC or Y-PSC will be correctly identified as having moderate to serious impairment in psychosocial functioning. The one child or adolescent "incorrectly" identified usually has at least mild impairment, although a small percentage of children and adolescents turn out to have very little or no impairment (e.g., an adequately functioning child or adolescent of an overly anxious parent). Data on PSC and Y-PSC negative screens indicate 95 percent accuracy, which, although statistically adequate, still means that 1 out of 20 children and adolescents rated as functioning adequately may actually be impaired. The inevitability of both false-positive and false-negative screens underscores the importance of experienced clinical judgment in interpreting PSC scores. Therefore, it is especially important for parents or other laypeople who administer the form to consult with a licensed professional if their child receives a PSC or Y-PSC positive score.

For more information, visit the Web site: http://psc.partners.org.

**REFERENCES**

Jellinek MS, Murphy JM, Little M, et al. 1999. Use of the Pediatric Symptom Checklist (PSC) to screen for psychosocial problems in pediatric primary care: A national feasibility study. *Archives of Pediatric and Adolescent Medicine* 153(3):254–260.

Jellinek MS, Murphy JM, Robinson J, et al. 1988. Pediatric Symptom Checklist: Screening school-age children for psychosocial dysfunction. *Journal of Pediatrics* 112(2):201–209. Web site: http://psc.partners.org.

Little M, Murphy JM, Jellinek MS, et al. 1994. Screening 4- and 5-year-old children for psychosocial dysfunction: A preliminary study with the Pediatric Symptom Checklist. *Journal of Developmental and Behavioral Pediatrics* 15:191–197.

Pagano M, Murphy JM, Pedersen M, et al. 1996. Screening for psychosocial problems in 4–5 year olds during routine EPSDT examinations: Validity and reliability in a Mexican-American sample. *Clinical Pediatrics* 35(3):139–146.

BRIGHT FUTURES ☀ TOOL FOR PROFESSIONALS

# Pediatric Symptom Checklist (PSC)

otional and physical health go together in children. Because parents are often the first to notice a problem with their
d's behavior, emotions, or learning, you may help your child get the best care possible by answering these questions.
se indicate which statement best describes your child.

**se mark under the heading that best describes your child:**

| | | Never | Sometimes | Often |
|---|---|---|---|---|
| Complains of aches and pains | 1 | | | |
| Spends more time alone | 2 | | | |
| Tires easily, has little energy | 3 | | | |
| Fidgety, unable to sit still | 4 | | | |
| Has trouble with teacher | 5 | | | |
| Less interested in school | 6 | | | |
| Acts as if driven by a motor | 7 | | | |
| Daydreams too much | 8 | | | |
| Distracted easily | 9 | | | |
| . Is afraid of new situations | 10 | | | |
| . Feels sad, unhappy | 11 | | | |
| . Is irritable, angry | 12 | | | |
| . Feels hopeless | 13 | | | |
| . Has trouble concentrating | 14 | | | |
| . Less interested in friends | 15 | | | |
| . Fights with other children | 16 | | | |
| . Absent from school | 17 | | | |
| . School grades dropping | 18 | | | |
| . Is down on him or herself | 19 | | | |
| . Visits the doctor with doctor finding nothing wrong | 20 | | | |
| . Has trouble sleeping | 21 | | | |
| . Worries a lot | 22 | | | |
| . Wants to be with you more than before | 23 | | | |
| . Feels he or she is bad | 24 | | | |
| . Takes unnecessary risks | 25 | | | |
| . Gets hurt frequently | 26 | | | |
| . Seems to be having less fun | 27 | | | |
| . Acts younger than children his or her age | 28 | | | |
| . Does not listen to rules | 29 | | | |
| . Does not show feelings | 30 | | | |
| . Does not understand other people's feelings | 31 | | | |
| . Teases others | 32 | | | |
| . Blames others for his or her troubles | 33 | | | |
| . Takes things that do not belong to him or her | 34 | | | |
| . Refuses to share | 35 | | | |

tal score _____

es your child have any emotional or behavioral problems for which she or he needs help?     ( ) N    ( ) Y
there any services that you would like your child to receive for these problems?     ( ) N    ( ) Y

s, what services?_____

www.brightfutures.org

# Pediatric Symptom Checklist—Youth Report (Y-PSC)

**Please mark under the heading that best fits you:**

|  |  | Never | Sometimes | Often |
|---|---|---|---|---|
| 1. Complain of aches or pains | 1 | | | |
| 2. Spend more time alone | 2 | | | |
| 3. Tire easily, little energy | 3 | | | |
| 4. Fidgety, unable to sit still | 4 | | | |
| 5. Have trouble with teacher | 5 | | | |
| 6. Less interested in school | 6 | | | |
| 7. Act as if driven by motor | 7 | | | |
| 8. Daydream too much | 8 | | | |
| 9. Distract easily | 9 | | | |
| 10. Are afraid of new situations | 10 | | | |
| 11. Feel sad, unhappy | 11 | | | |
| 12. Are irritable, angry | 12 | | | |
| 13. Feel hopeless | 13 | | | |
| 14. Have trouble concentrating | 14 | | | |
| 15. Less interested in friends | 15 | | | |
| 16. Fight with other children | 16 | | | |
| 17. Absent from school | 17 | | | |
| 18. School grades dropping | 18 | | | |
| 19. Down on yourself | 19 | | | |
| 20. Visit doctor with doctor finding nothing wrong | 20 | | | |
| 21. Have trouble sleeping | 21 | | | |
| 22. Worry a lot | 22 | | | |
| 23. Want to be with parent more than before | 23 | | | |
| 24. Feel that you are bad | 24 | | | |
| 25. Take unnecessary risks | 25 | | | |
| 26. Get hurt frequently | 26 | | | |
| 27. Seem to be having less fun | 27 | | | |
| 28. Act younger than children your age | 28 | | | |
| 29. Do not listen to rules | 29 | | | |
| 30. Do not show feelings | 30 | | | |
| 31. Do not understand other people's feelings | 31 | | | |
| 32. Tease others | 32 | | | |
| 33. Blame others for your troubles | 33 | | | |
| 34. Take things that do not belong to you | 34 | | | |
| 35. Refuse to share | 35 | | | |

# Vanderbilt Assessment Scale for ADHD

The Vanderbilt Assessment Scale for attention-deficit/hyperactivity disorder (ADHD) is a diagnosis-specific screening tool designed to aid in the assessment and management of children aged 6 to 12 with ADHD. It is reproduced on the next page and is available online at www.nichq.org/childrens-health /adhd/resources/vanderbilt-assessment-scales. It is available in long (assessment) and short (treatment monitoring) versions for both parents and teachers. The long versions include an assessment of potential comorbidities.

# NICHQ Vanderbilt Assessment Scale: Parent Informant

Today's Date: 08-25-15

Child's Name: _____

Child's Date of Birth: _____

Parent's Name: _____

Parent's Phone Number: _____

**Directions: Each rating should be considered in the context of what is appropriate for the age of your child. When completing this form, please think about your child's behaviors in the past 6 months.**

**Is this evaluation based on a time when the child**

○ was on medication     ○ was not on medication     ○ not sure?

| Symptoms | Never | Occasionally | Often | Very Often |
| --- | --- | --- | --- | --- |
| 1. Does not pay attention to details or makes careless mistakes with, for example, homework | ○ | ○ | ○ | ○ |
| 2. Has difficulty keeping attention to what needs to be done | ○ | ○ | ○ | ○ |
| 3. Does not seem to listen when spoken to directly | ○ | ○ | ○ | ○ |
| 4. Does not follow through when given directions and fails to finish activities (not due to refusal or failure to understand) | ○ | ○ | ○ | ○ |
| 5. Has difficulty organizing tasks and activities | ○ | ○ | ○ | ○ |
| 6. Avoids, dislikes, or does not want to start tasks that require ongoing mental effort | ○ | ○ | ○ | ○ |
| 7. Loses things necessary for tasks or activities (toys, assignments, pencils, books) | ○ | ○ | ○ | ○ |
| 8. Is easily distracted by noises or other stimuli | ○ | ○ | ○ | ○ |
| 9. Is forgetful in daily activities | ○ | ○ | ○ | ○ |
| 10. Fidgets with hands or feet or squirms in seat | ○ | ○ | ○ | ○ |
| 11. Leaves seat when remaining seated is expected | ○ | ○ | ○ | ○ |
| 12. Runs about or climbs too much when remaining seated is expected | ○ | ○ | ○ | ○ |
| 13. Has difficulty playing or beginning quiet play activities | ○ | ○ | ○ | ○ |
| 14. Is "on the go" or often acts as if "driven by a motor" | ○ | ○ | ○ | ○ |
| 15. Talks too much | ○ | ○ | ○ | ○ |
| 16. Blurts out answers before questions have been completed | ○ | ○ | ○ | ○ |
| 17. Has difficulty waiting his or her turn | ○ | ○ | ○ | ○ |
| 18. Interrupts or intrudes in on others' conversations and/or activities | ○ | ○ | ○ | ○ |

For Office Use Only 2 & 3s: 0

For Office Use Only 2 & 3s: 0

🏃🏃🏃🏃 NICHQ Vanderbilt Assessment Scale: Parent Informant

| Symptoms (continued) | Never | Occasionally | Often | Very Often | |
|---|---|---|---|---|---|
| 19. Argues with adults | O | O | O | O | |
| 20. Loses temper | O | O | O | O | |
| 21. Actively defies or refuses to go along with adults' requests or rules | O | O | O | O | |
| 22. Deliberately annoys people | O | O | O | O | |
| 23. Blames others for his or her mistakes or misbehaviors | O | O | O | O | |
| 24. Is touchy or easily annoyed by others | O | O | O | O | |
| 25. Is angry or resentful | O | O | O | O | |
| 26. Is spiteful and wants to get even | O | O | O | O | For Office Use Only 2 & 3s: 0 /8 |
| 27. Bullies, threatens, or intimidates others | O | O | O | O | |
| 28. Starts physical fights | O | O | O | O | |
| 29. Lies to get out of trouble or to avoid obligations (ie, "cons" others) | O | O | O | O | |
| 30. Is truant from school (skips school) without permission | O | O | O | O | |
| 31. Is physically cruel to people | O | O | O | O | |
| 32. Has stolen things that have value | O | O | O | O | |
| 33. Deliberately destroys others' property | O | O | O | O | |
| 34. Has used a weapon that can cause serious harm (bat, knife, brick, gun) | O | O | O | O | |
| 35. Is physically cruel to animals | O | O | O | O | |
| 36. Has deliberately set fires to cause damage | O | O | O | O | |
| 37. Has broken into someone else's home, business, or car | O | O | O | O | |
| 38. Has stayed out at night without permission | O | O | O | O | |
| 39. Has run away from home overnight | O | O | O | O | |
| 40. Has forced someone into sexual activity | O | O | O | O | For Office Use Only 2&3s: 0 /14 |
| 41. Is fearful, anxious, or worried | O | O | O | O | |
| 42. Is afraid to try new things for fear of making mistakes | O | O | O | O | |
| 43. Feels worthless or inferior | O | O | O | O | |
| 44. Blames self for problems, feels guilty | O | O | O | O | |
| 45. Feels lonely, unwanted, or unloved; complains that "no one loves him or her" | O | O | O | O | |
| 46. Is sad, unhappy, or depressed | O | O | O | O | |
| 47. Is self-conscious or easily embarrassed | O | O | O | O | For Office Use Only 2 & 3s: 0 /7 |

| Performance | Excellent | Above Average | Average | Somewhat of a Problem | Problematic | |
|---|---|---|---|---|---|---|
| 48. Reading | O | O | O | O | O | |
| 49. Writing | O | O | O | O | O | For Office Use Only 4s: 0 /3 |
| 50. Mathematics | O | O | O | O | O | For Office Use Only 5s: 0 /3 |
| 51. Relationship with parents | O | O | O | O | O | |
| 52. Relationship with siblings | O | O | O | O | O | |
| 53. Relationship with peers | O | O | O | O | O | For Office Use Only 4s: 0 /4 |
| 54. Participation in organized activities (eg, teams) | O | O | O | O | O | For Office Use Only 5s: 0 /4 |

## Other Conditions

**Tic Behaviors:** To the best of your knowledge, please indicate if this child displays the following behaviors:

1. **Motor Tics:** Rapid, repetitive movements such as eye blinking, grimacing, nose twitching, head jerks, shoulder shrugs, arm jerks, body jerks, or rapid kicks.

   ☐ No tics present.  ☐ Yes, they occur nearly every day but go unnoticed by most people.  ☐ Yes, noticeable tics occur nearly every day.

2. **Phonic (Vocal) Tics:** Repetitive noises including but not limited to throat clearing, coughing, whistling, sniffing, snorting, screeching, barking, grunting, or repetition of words or short phrases.

   ☐ No tics present.  ☐ Yes, they occur nearly every day but go unnoticed by most people.  ☐ Yes, noticeable tics occur nearly every day.

3. If **YES** to 1 or 2, do these tics interfere with the child's activities (like reading, writing, walking, talking, or eating)?  ☐ No  ☐ Yes

**Previous Diagnosis and Treatment:** To the best of your knowledge, please answer the following questions:

| | | |
|---|---|---|
| 1. Has your child been diagnosed with a tic disorder or Tourette syndrome? | ☐ No | ☐ Yes |
| 2. Is your child on medication for a tic disorder or Tourette syndrome? | ☐ No | ☐ Yes |
| 3. Has your child been diagnosed with depression? | ☐ No | ☐ Yes |
| 4. Is your child on medication for depression? | ☐ No | ☐ Yes |
| 5. Has your child been diagnosed with an anxiety disorder? | ☐ No | ☐ Yes |
| 6. Is your child on medication for an anxiety disorder? | ☐ No | ☐ Yes |
| 7. Has your child been diagnosed with a learning or language disorder? | ☐ No | ☐ Yes |

**Comments:**

🏃🏃🏃🏃 NICHQ Vanderbilt Assessment Scale: Parent Informant

---

**For Office Use Only**

Total number of questions scored 2 or 3 in questions 1–9: _____

Total number of questions scored 2 or 3 in questions 10–18: _____

Total number of questions scored 2 or 3 in questions 19–26: _____

Total number of questions scored 2 or 3 in questions 27–40: _____

Total number of questions scored 2 or 3 in questions 41–47: _____

Total number of questions scored 4 in questions 48–50: _____

Total number of questions scored 5 in questions 48–50: _____

Total number of questions scored 4 in questions 51–54: _____

Total number of questions scored 5 in questions 51–54: _____

---

Adapted from the Vanderbilt Rating Scales developed by Mark L. Wolraich, MD.

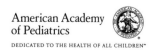

American Academy
of Pediatrics
DEDICATED TO THE HEALTH OF ALL CHILDREN™

QuIIN
Quality Improvement
Innovation Network
A program of the American Academy of Pediatrics

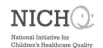

NICHQ
National Initiative for
Children's Healthcare Quality

ADHD ꙮ CARING FOR CHILDREN WITH ADHD: A RESOURCE TOOLKIT FOR CLINICIANS, 2ND EDITION

# Scoring Instructions for NICHQ Vanderbilt Assessment Scales

## Baseline Assessment

The validation studies for the NICHQ Vanderbilt Assessment Scales were for the 6- to 12-year-old age group. However, to the extent that they collect information to establish *Diagnostic and Statistical Manual of Mental Disorders, Fifth Edition (DSM-5)* criteria, they are applicable to other groups, particularly preschoolers, where they have identified that *DSM-5* criteria are still appropriate.

These scales should *not* be used alone to make a diagnosis of ADHD without confirming and elaborating the information with interviews with at least the primary caregivers (usually parents) and patients. You must take into consideration information from multiple sources. Scores of 2 or 3 on a single symptom question reflect *often-occurring* behaviors. Scores of 4 or 5 on performance questions reflect problems in performance.

The initial assessment scales, parent and teacher, have 2 components: symptom assessment and impairment in performance. On both parent and teacher initial scales, the symptom assessment screens for symptoms that meet criteria for inattentive (items 1–9) and hyperactive (items 10–18) attention-deficit/hyperactivity disorder (ADHD).

### Scoring for Diagnostic Purposes

To meet *DSM-5* criteria for the diagnosis, one must have at least 6 positive responses to the inattentive 9 or hyperactive 9 core symptoms, or both. A positive response is a 2 or 3 (often, very often) (you could draw a line straight down the page and count the positive answers in each subsegment). There is a place to record the number of positives in each subsegment.

The initial scales have symptom screens for 3 other comorbidities: oppositional-defiant disorder, conduct disorder, and anxiety/depression. (The initial teacher scale also screens for learning disabilities.) These are screened by the number of positive responses in each of the segments. The specific item sets and numbers of positives required for each comorbid symptom screen set are detailed below and on the next page.

The second section of the scale has a set of performance measures, scored 1 to 5, with 4 and 5 being somewhat of a problem/problematic. To meet criteria for ADHD there must be at least 2 items of the performance set in which the child scores a 4, or 1 item of the performance set in which the child scores a 5; ie, there must be impairment, not just symptoms, to meet diagnostic criteria. The sheet has a place to record the number of positives (4s, 5s).

### Scoring to Monitor Symptom and Performance Improvement

For the purposes of tracking symptoms and symptom severity, calculate the mean response for each subsegment of the ADHD symptom assessment screen items (inattentive 9 and hyperactive 9). To calculate the mean responses, first total the responses (0s, 1s, 2s, and 3s) from each item within the inattentive subsegment (items 1–9) and divide by the number of items that received a response. For example, if a parent only provided responses to 7 of the first 9 items, the responses would be totaled and divided by 7. Follow the same calculation instructions for the hyperactive subsegment (items 10–18).

| Parent Assessment Scale | Teacher Assessment Scale |
|---|---|
| **Predominantly Inattentive subtype**<br>• Must score a 2 or 3 on 6 out of 9 items on questions 1–9.<br><u>AND</u><br>• Score a 4 on at least 2, or 5 on at least 1, of the performance questions 48–54. | **Predominantly Inattentive subtype**<br>• Must score a 2 or 3 on 6 out of 9 items on questions 1–9.<br><u>AND</u><br>• Score a 4 on at least 2, or 5 on at least 1, of the performance questions 36–43. |
| **Predominantly Hyperactive/Impulsive subtype**<br>• Must score a 2 or 3 on 6 out of 9 items on questions 10–18.<br><u>AND</u><br>• Score a 4 on at least 2, or 5 on at least 1, of the performance questions 48–54. | **Predominantly Hyperactive/Impulsive subtype**<br>• Must score a 2 or 3 on 6 out of 9 items on questions 10–18.<br><u>AND</u><br>• Score a 4 on at least 2, or 5 on at least 1, of the performance questions 36–43. |
| **ADHD Combined Inattention/Hyperactivity**<br>• Requires the criteria on Inattentive <u>AND</u> Hyperactive/Impulsive subtypes | **ADHD Combined Inattention/Hyperactivity**<br>• Requires the criteria on Inattentive <u>AND</u> Hyperactive/Impulsive subtypes |
| **Oppositional-Defiant Disorder**<br>• Must score a 2 or 3 on 4 out of 8 behaviors on questions 19–26.<br><u>AND</u><br>• Score a 4 on at least 2, or 5 on at least 1, of the performance questions 48–54. | **Oppositional-Defiant/Conduct Disorder**<br>• Must score a 2 or 3 on 3 out of 10 items on questions 19–28.<br><u>AND</u><br>• Score a 4 on at least 2, or 5 on at least 1, of the performance questions 36–43. |
| **Conduct Disorder**<br>• Must score a 2 or 3 on 3 out of 14 behaviors on questions 27–40.<br><u>AND</u><br>• Score a 4 on at least 2, or 5 on at least 1, of the performance questions 48–54. | |

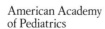 Scoring Instructions for NICHQ Vanderbilt Assessment Scales

| Parent Assessment Scale | Teacher Assessment Scale |
|---|---|
| **Anxiety/Depression**<br>• Must score a 2 or 3 on 3 out of 7 behaviors on questions 41–47.<br>AND<br>• Score a 4 on at least 2, or 5 on at least 1, of the performance questions 48–54. | **Anxiety/Depression**<br>• Must score a 2 or 3 on 3 out of 7 items on questions 29–35.<br>AND<br>• Score a 4 on at least 2, or 5 on at least 1, of the performance questions 36–43.<br><br>**Learning Disabilities**<br>• Must score a 4 on both, or 5 on 1, of questions 36 and 38. |

## Follow-up Assessment

### Scoring for Diagnostic Purposes

The parent and teacher follow-up scales have the first 18 core ADHD symptoms and the comorbid symptoms oppositional-defiant (parent) and oppositional-defiant/conduct (teacher) disorders. The Performance section has the same performance items and impairment assessment as the initial scales; it is followed by a side-effect reporting scale that can be used to assess and monitor the presence of adverse reactions to prescribed medications, if any.

Scoring the follow-up scales involves tracking inattentive items 1–9) and hyperactive (items 10–18) ADHD, as well as the

aforementioned comorbidities, as measures of improvement over time with treatment.

### Scoring to Monitor Symptom and Performance Improvement

To determine the score for follow-up, calculate the mean response for each of the ADHD subsegments. Compare the mean response from the follow-up inattentive subsegment (items 1–9) to the mean response from the inattentive subsegment that was calculated at baseline assessment. Conduct the same comparison for the mean responses for the hyperactive subsegment (items 10–18) taken at follow-up and baseline.

| Parent Assessment Scale | Teacher Assessment Scale |
|---|---|
| **Predominantly Inattentive subtype**<br>• Must score a 2 or 3 on 6 out of 9 items on questions 1–9.<br>AND<br>• Score a 4 on at least 2, or 5 on at least 1, of the performance questions 27–33. | **Predominantly Inattentive subtype**<br>• Must score a 2 or 3 on 6 out of 9 items on questions 1–9.<br>AND<br>• Score a 4 on at least 2, or 5 on at least 1, of the performance questions 29–36. |
| **Predominantly Hyperactive/Impulsive subtype**<br>• Must score a 2 or 3 on 6 out of 9 items on questions 10–18.<br>AND<br>• Score a 4 on at least 2, or 5 on at least 1, of the performance questions 27–33. | **Predominantly Hyperactive/Impulsive subtype**<br>• Must score a 2 or 3 on 6 out of 9 items on questions 10–18.<br>AND<br>• Score a 4 on at least 2, or 5 on at least 1, of the performance questions 29–36. |
| **ADHD Combined Inattention/Hyperactivity**<br>• Requires the criteria on Inattentive AND Hyperactive/Impulsive subtypes | **ADHD Combined Inattention/Hyperactivity**<br>• Requires the criteria on Inattentive AND Hyperactive/Impulsive subtypes |
| **Oppositional-Defiant Disorder**<br>• Must score a 2 or 3 on 4 out of 8 behaviors on questions 19–26.<br>AND<br>• Score a 4 on at least 2, or 5 on at least 1, of the performance questions 27–33. | **Oppositional-Defiant/Conduct Disorder**<br>• Must score a 2 or 3 on 3 out of 10 items on questions 19–28.<br>AND<br>• Score a 4 on at least 2, or 5 on at least 1, of the performance questions 29–36. |

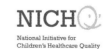

American Academy of Pediatrics
DEDICATED TO THE HEALTH OF ALL CHILDREN™

QuIIN
Quality Improvement Innovation Network
A program of the American Academy of Pediatrics

NICHQ
National Initiative for Children's Healthcare Quality

# Screen for Child Anxiety Related Disorders

The Screen for Child Anxiety Related Disorders (SCARED) is a diagnosis-specific tool designed to aid in the assessment and management of children aged 8 and older with anxiety. It is reproduced on the next page and is available at http://psychiatry.pitt.edu/sites/default/files/Documents/assessments/SCARED%20Child.pdf. Parent and teacher versions are available. Subscales include generalized anxiety, social anxiety, separation anxiety, school avoidance, and panic attack symptoms.

# Screen for Child Anxiety Related Disorders (SCARED)
## CHILD Version—Page 1 of 2 (to be filled out by the CHILD)

Developed by Boris Birmaher, M.D., Suneeta Khetarpal, M.D., Marlane Cully, M.Ed., David Brent, M.D., and Sandra McKenzie, Ph.D., Western Psychiatric Institute and Clinic, University of Pittsburgh *(October, 1995)*. *E-mail:* birmaherb@upmc.edu

See: Birmaher, B., Brent, D. A., Chiappetta, L., Bridge, J., Monga, S., & Baugher, M. (1999). Psychometric properties of the Screen for Child Anxiety Related Emotional Disorders (SCARED): a replication study. *Journal of the American Academy of Child and Adolescent Psychiatry, 38*(10), 1230–6.

Name: _____     Date: _____

**Directions**:
Below is a list of sentences that describe how people feel. Read each phrase and decide if it is "Not True or Hardly Ever True" or "Somewhat True or Sometimes True" or "Very True or Often True" for you. Then, for each sentence, fill in one circle that corresponds to the response that seems to describe you *for the last 3 months*.

| | 0<br>Not True<br>or Hardly<br>Ever True | 1<br>Somewhat<br>True or<br>Sometimes<br>True | 2<br>Very True<br>or Often<br>True | |
|---|:---:|:---:|:---:|---|
| 1. When I feel frightened, it is hard to breathe | O | O | O | PN |
| 2. I get headaches when I am at school. | O | O | O | SH |
| 3. I don't like to be with people I don't know well. | O | O | O | SC |
| 4. I get scared if I sleep away from home. | O | O | O | SP |
| 5. I worry about other people liking me. | O | O | O | GD |
| 6. When I get frightened, I feel like passing out. | O | O | O | PN |
| 7. I am nervous. | O | O | O | GD |
| 8. I follow my mother or father wherever they go. | O | O | O | SP |
| 9. People tell me that I look nervous. | O | O | O | PN |
| 10. I feel nervous with people I don't know well. | O | O | O | SC |
| 11. I get stomachaches at school. | O | O | O | SH |
| 12. When I get frightened, I feel like I am going crazy. | O | O | O | PN |
| 13. I worry about sleeping alone. | O | O | O | SP |
| 14. I worry about being as good as other kids. | O | O | O | GD |
| 15. When I get frightened, I feel like things are not real. | O | O | O | PN |
| 16. I have nightmares about something bad happening to my parents. | O | O | O | SP |
| 17. I worry about going to school. | O | O | O | SH |
| 18. When I get frightened, my heart beats fast. | O | O | O | PN |
| 19. I get shaky. | O | O | O | PN |
| 20. I have nightmares about something bad happening to me. | O | O | O | SP |

## Screen for Child Anxiety Related Disorders (SCARED)
### CHILD Version—Page 2 of 2 (to be filled out by the CHILD)

| | 0<br>Not True<br>or Hardly<br>Ever True | 1<br>Somewhat<br>True or<br>Sometimes<br>True | 2<br>Very True<br>or Often<br>True | |
|---|---|---|---|---|
| 21. I worry about things working out for me. | O | O | O | GD |
| 22. When I get frightened, I sweat a lot. | O | O | O | PN |
| 23. I am a worrier. | O | O | O | GD |
| 24. I get really frightened for no reason at all. | O | O | O | PN |
| 25. I am afraid to be alone in the house. | O | O | O | SP |
| 26. It is hard for me to talk with people I don't know well. | O | O | O | SC |
| 27. When I get frightened, I feel like I am choking. | O | O | O | PN |
| 28. People tell me that I worry too much. | O | O | O | GD |
| 29. I don't like to be away from my family. | O | O | O | SP |
| 30. I am afraid of having anxiety (or panic) attacks. | O | O | O | PN |
| 31. I worry that something bad might happen to my parents. | O | O | O | SP |
| 32. I feel shy with people I don't know well. | O | O | O | SC |
| 33. I worry about what is going to happen in the future. | O | O | O | GD |
| 34. When I get frightened, I feel like throwing up. | O | O | O | PN |
| 35. I worry about how well I do things. | O | O | O | GD |
| 36. I am scared to go to school. | O | O | O | SH |
| 37. I worry about things that have already happened. | O | O | O | GD |
| 38. When I get frightened, I feel dizzy. | O | O | O | PN |
| 39. I feel nervous when I am with other children or adults and I have to do something while they watch me (for example: read aloud, speak, play a game, play a sport). | O | O | O | SC |
| 40. I feel nervous when I am going to parties, dances, or any place where there will be people that I don't know well. | O | O | O | SC |
| 41. I am shy. | O | O | O | SC |

**SCORING:**

A total score of ≥ 25 may indicate the presence of an **Anxiety Disorder**. Scores higher than 30 are more specific. | TOTAL = |

A score of 7 for items 1, 6, 9, 12, 15, 18, 19, 22, 24, 27, 30, 34, 38 may indicate **Panic Disorder** or **Significant Somatic Symptoms.** | PN = |

A score of 9 for items 5, 7, 14, 21, 23, 28, 33, 35, 37 may indicate **Generalized Anxiety Disorder**. | GD = |

A score of 5 for items 4, 8, 13, 16, 20, 25, 29, 31 may indicate **Separation Anxiety SOC.** | SP = |

A score of 8 for items 3, 10, 26, 32, 39, 40, 41 may indicate **Social Anxiety Disorder.** | SC = |

A score of 3 for items 2, 11, 17, 36 may indicate **Significant School Avoidance.** | SH = |

*For children ages 8 to 11, it is recommended that the clinician explain all questions, or have the child answer the questionnaire sitting with an adult in case they have any questions.*

*The SCARED is available at no cost at www.wpic.pitt.edu/research under tools and assessments, or at www.pediatric.bipolar.pitt.edu under instruments*

# Patient Health Questionnaire-9 Modified for Teens

The Patient Health Questionnaire-9 (PHQ-9) Modified for Teens is a diagnosis-specific screening tool designed to assess for symptoms of depression in teenagers. It is reproduced on the next page and is available online at www.thereachinstitute.org/images/GLAD-PCToolkit_V2_2010.pdf. It also provides a brief assessment of suicidal ideation.

# PHQ-9: Modified for Teens

Name: _____ Clinician: _____ Date: _____

**Instructions:** How often have you been bothered by each of the following symptoms during the past **two weeks**? For each symptom put an **"X"** in the box beneath the answer that best describes how you have been feeling.

|  | (0)<br>Not At All | (1)<br>Several Days | (2)<br>More Than Half the Days | (3)<br>Nearly Every Day |
|---|---|---|---|---|
| 1. Feeling down, depressed, irritable, or hopeless? |  |  |  |  |
| 2. Little interest or pleasure in doing things? |  |  |  |  |
| 3. Trouble falling asleep, staying asleep, or sleeping too much? |  |  |  |  |
| 4. Poor appetite, weight loss, or overeating? |  |  |  |  |
| 5. Feeling tired, or having little energy? |  |  |  |  |
| 6. Feeling bad about yourself – or feeling that you are a failure, or that you have let yourself or your family down? |  |  |  |  |
| 7. Trouble concentrating on things like school work, reading, or watching TV? |  |  |  |  |
| 8. Moving or speaking so slowly that other people could have noticed?<br><br>Or the opposite – being so fidgety or restless that you were moving around a lot more than usual? |  |  |  |  |
| 9. Thoughts that you would be better off dead, or of hurting yourself in some way? |  |  |  |  |

In the **past year** have you felt depressed or sad most days, even if you felt okay sometimes?
[ ] Yes          [ ] No

If you are experiencing any of the problems on this form, how **difficult** have these problems made it for you to do your work, take care of things at home or get along with other people?

[ ] Not difficult at all      [ ] Somewhat difficult      [ ] Very difficult      [ ] Extremely difficult

---

Has there been a time in the **past month** when you have had serious thoughts about ending your life?
[ ] Yes          [ ] No

Have you **EVER**, in your WHOLE LIFE, tried to kill yourself or made a suicide attempt?
[ ] Yes          [ ] No

*\*\*If you have had thoughts that you would be better off dead or of hurting yourself in some way, please discuss this with your Health Care Clinician, go to a hospital emergency room or call 911.*

**Office use only:**     **Severity score:** _____

Modified with permission by the GLAD-PC team from the PHQ-9 (Spitzer, Williams, & Kroenke, 1999), Revised PHQ-A (Johnson, 2002), and the CDS (DISC Development Group, 2000)

Used with the permission of the REACH Institute (www.thereachinstitute.org).

# Scoring the PHQ-9 modified for Teens

Scoring the PHQ-9 modified for teens is easy but involves thinking about several different aspects of depression.

To use the PHQ-9 as a diagnostic aid for Major Depressive Disorder:
- Questions 1 and/or 2 need to be endorsed as a "2" or "3"
- Need five or more positive symptoms (positive is defined by a "2" or "3" in questions 1-8 and by a "1", "2", or "3" in question 9).
- The functional impairment question (How difficult....) needs to be rated at least as "somewhat difficult."

To use the PHQ-9 to screen for all types of depression or other mental illness:
- All positive answers (positive is defined by a "2" or "3" in questions 1-8 and by a "1", "2", or "3" in question 9) should be followed up by interview.
- A total PHQ-9 score $\geq$ 10 (see below for instructions on how to obtain a total score) has a good sensitivity and specificity for MDD.

To use the PHQ-9 to aid in the diagnosis of dysthymia:
- The dysthymia question (In the past year...) should be endorsed as "yes."

To use the PHQ-9 to screen for suicide risk:
- All positive answers to question 9 as well as the two additional suicide items MUST be followed up by a clinical interview.

To use the PHQ-9 to obtain a total score and assess depressive severity:
- Add up the numbers endorsed for questions 1-9 and obtain a total score.
- See Table below:

| Total Score | Depression Severity |
|---|---|
| 0-4 | No or Minimal depression |
| 5-9 | Mild depression |
| 10-14 | Moderate depression |
| 15-19 | Moderately severe depression |
| 20-27 | Severe depression |

# Other Assessment and Monitoring Tools

## Strengths and Difficulties Questionnaire

The Strengths and Difficulties Questionnaire (SDQ) is a general screening tool for identifying emotional and behavioral concerns in youths aged 2 to 17 years. Parent, teacher, and self-report versions are available online at www.sdqinfo.com. Questions highlight challenges as well as strengths. Versions with and without symptom effect are available. Subscales include emotional problems, conduct problems, hyperactivity, and peer problems.

## Pediatric Sleep Log

The pediatric sleep log is a tool designed to help families track sleep patterns to look for opportunities to improve sleep quality. See more at www.brightfutures.org/mentalhealth/pdf/families/ec/diary.pdf.

## Tools to Identify Children Exposed to Violence

The "Tools to Identify Children Exposed to Violence" Web page provides a summary of screening tools that can be helpful in identifying children exposed to trauma. It is available at www.aap.org/en-us/advocacy-and-policy/aap-health-initiatives/Medical-Home-for-Children-and-Adolescents-Exposed-to-Violence/Pages/Diagnostic-Tools.aspx.

## Safe Environment for Every Kid Questionnaire

The Safe Environment for Every Kid (SEEK) questionnaire is a brief screening tool designed to identify potential environment needs and safety concerns. It is available at www.uspreventiveservicestaskforce.org/Home/GetFileByID/859.

## CRAFFT Screening Tool

The CRAFFT (car, relax, alone, forget, friends, trouble) Screening Tool is designed to identify youths at risk for problems related to substance use. It is available at www.ceasar-boston.org/CRAFFT/index.php.

## Abnormal Involuntary Movement Scale

The Abnormal Involuntary Movement Scale (AIMS) is designed to systematically assess for the presence of involuntary movements that may be associated with antipsychotic medications. The scale is available at

http://imaging.ubmmedica.com/all/editorial/psychiatrictimes/pdfs/clinical
-scales-aims-form.pdf. A demonstration of the examination procedure is
available at http://imaging.ubmmedica.com/all/editorial/psychiatrictimes
/pdfs/clinical-scales-aims-instructions.pdf.

## Barnes Akathisia Rating Scale

The Barnes Akathisia Rating Scale is a 4-item tool used to assess the
presence and severity of drug-induced akathisia. It is available at
http://keltymentalhealth.ca/sites/default/files/BARS.pdf.

# Treatment Tools

## Treatment of Maladaptive Aggression in Youth

Treatment of Maladaptive Aggression in Youth (T-MAY) provides guidelines
for management and treatment of maladaptive aggression in the areas of
family engagement, assessment and diagnosis, and initial management. It is
appropriate for use by primary care clinicians and mental health providers.
It was developed by a steering group of national experts and published as
a supplement in *Pediatrics*. Part 1 can be accessed at http://pediatrics
.aappublications.org/content/129/6/e1562.full?sid=2c6d87cb-2928-4269
-86e2-e4caae4ff805, and Part 2 can be accessed at http://pediatrics
.aappublications.org/content/129/6/e1577.full?sid=2c6d87cb-2928-4269
-86e2-e4caae4ff805.

## HELP

Pediatric primary care clinicians, when presented with a child's mental health
problem, can often take steps to address parents' distress and children's
symptoms, regardless of the specific diagnosis. They can employ effective
family-centered techniques known as common factors, so-called because
they are common factors in a number of evidence-based interventions. These
can be represented by the mnemonic HELP: Hope, Empathy, Language,
Loyalty, Permission, Partnership, Plan.

A full description of HELP can be found in *Addressing Mental Health
Concerns in Primary Care: A Clinicians Toolkit*. See more at www.aap.org
/en-us/advocacy-and-policy/aap-health-initiatives/Mental-Health/Pages
/Addressing-Mental-Health-Concerns-in-Primary-Care-A-Clinicians
-Toolkit.aspx#sthash.ndeXJpGp.dpuf.

## Generic or Common Factors Intervention Tool

The Generic or Common Factors Intervention tool describes important strategies to improve communication and family engagement: hope, empathy, language, loyalty, and plan. It can be found in *Addressing Mental Health Concerns in Primary Care: A Clinicians Toolkit.* See more at www.aap.org /en-us/advocacy-and-policy/aap-health-initiatives/Mental-Health/Pages /Addressing-Mental-Health-Concerns-in-Primary-Care-A-Clinicians-Toolkit .aspx#sthash.ndeXJpGp.dpuf.

## Patient Counseling Section in US FDA Package Insert

To see an example of the Patient Counseling Information section for fluoxetine, see page 24 of the insert located at www.accessdata.fda.gov/drugsatfda _docs/label/2011/018936s091lbl.pdf.

# Practice Readiness and Sources of Specialty Services Tools

## Mental Health Practice Readiness Inventory

The practice readiness inventory is a questionnaire designed to help primary care practices determine their level of readiness to address mental health concerns. It can be found in *Addressing Mental Health Concerns in Primary Care: A Clinicians Toolkit.* See more at www.aap.org/en-us/advocacy-and -policy/aap-health-initiatives/Mental-Health/Pages/Addressing-Mental -Health-Concerns-in-Primary-Care-A-Clinicians-Toolkit.aspx#sthash .ndeXJpGp.dpuf.

## Sources of Specialty Services for Children With Mental Health Problems and Their Families

The Sources of Specialty Services for Children With Mental Health Problems and Their Families handout summarizes key mental health referral services for children and adolescents. It can be found in *Addressing Mental Health Concerns in Primary Care: A Clinicians Toolkit.* See more at www.aap.org /en-us/advocacy-and-policy/aap-health-initiatives/Mental-Health/Pages /Addressing-Mental-Health-Concerns-in-Primary-Care-A-Clinicians-Toolkit .aspx#sthash.ndeXJpGp.dpuf.

# Resources for Clinicians

## American Academy of Pediatrics

### "Mental Health Initiatives" Web Page

The "Mental Health Initiatives" Web page (www.aap.org/en-us/advocacy
-and-policy/aap-health-initiatives/Mental-Health/Pages/default.aspx) contains a number of tools and resources for practitioners caring for children
with mental health concerns.

### Toolkits

- *Addressing Mental Health Concerns in Primary Care: A Clinicians Toolkit*
  (www.aap.org/en-us/advocacy-and-policy/aap-health-initiatives
  /Mental-Health/Pages/Addressing-Mental-Health-Concerns-in-Primary
  -Care-A-Clinicians-Toolkit.aspx#sthash.ndeXJpGp.dpuf)
- *Caring for Children with ADHD: A Resource Toolkit for Clinicians*
  (https://www.aap.org/en-us/professional-resources/practice-support
  /quality-improvement/Quality-Improvement-Innovation-Networks
  /Pages/Guidelines-and-Tools-to-Improve-Care-for-Children-with
  -ADHD-Improvement-Project.aspx)

### Clinical Practice Guidelines for ADHD

The "ADHD: Clinical Practice Guideline for the Diagnosis, Evaluation,
and Treatment of Attention-Deficit/Hyperactivity Disorder in Children and
Adolescents" can be found at http://pediatrics.aappublications.org
/content/128/5/1007.full.pdf+html.

## "Enhancing Pediatric Mental Health Care"

This report from the Task Force on Mental Health can be found at http://pediatrics.aappublications.org/content/125/Supplement_3.toc.

# Neuroscience-Based Nomenclature App

The Neuroscience-Based Nomenclature app provides useful information about all 108 psychotropic medications that are available in the world, organized by 11 pharmacologic domains and 11 mechanisms of action.

- Apple: https://itunes.apple.com/us/app/nbn-neuroscience-based -nomenclature/id927272449?mt=8
- Android: https://play.google.com/store/apps/details?id=il.co.inmanage .nbnomenclature&hl=en

# National Network of Child Psychiatry Access Programs

The National Network of Child Psychiatry Access Programs is a collaboration of about 30 US state programs that provide varying levels of child psychiatry collaboration and consultation regarding mental health to pediatric primary care clinicians (www.nncpap.org).

# Training Resources for Clinicians

## The REACH Institute

The REACH Institute's mission is to transform children's health services by empowering their care professionals (ie, physicians, therapists, parents, and teachers) to know and use the most effective methods for identifying and assisting children with mental health conditions.

REACH (www.thereachinstitute.org) offers interactive, sustained coaching programs to primary care physicians, behavioral health care professionals, parent advocates, and educators. Specific programs include the Mini-Fellowship in Primary Pediatric Psychopharmacology, Child and Adolescent Training Institute for Evidence-Based Psychotherapies, and Parent Empowerment Programs designed for parents navigating mental health care systems, juvenile justice, and child welfare.

The Primary Pediatric Psychopharmacology Program is REACH's signature program. Through it, primary care medical professionals learn 4 essential skills: how to (1) assess and diagnose children with common mental health problems (eg, depression and anxiety disorders, attention-deficit/hyperactivity disorder [ADHD]); (2) ascertain the presence of more severe conditions that warrant referral to mental health specialists (eg, bipolar disorder, psychosis, or complex comorbid conditions); (3) form a comprehensive treatment plan (including identifying psychotherapy resources); and (4) safely and effectively use psychiatric medications to treat children and adolescents with ADHD, depression, anxiety disorders, and related conditions. The program includes an interactive 16-hour workshop (delivered over 3 days) and 6 months of ongoing case-based consultation with a child psychiatrist and primary care physician selected from REACH's nationally known pediatric psychopharmacology faculty.

# American Academy of Pediatrics

## Implementing Mental Health Priorities in Practice Videos

The *Implementing Mental Health Priorities in Practice* videos provide examples of the use of motivational interviewing to approach common mental health concerns in pediatrics (www.aap.org/en-us/advocacy-and-policy /aap-health-initiatives/Mental-Health/Pages/introduction.aspx).

## Mental Health Leadership Work Group Residency Curriculum, Module 2: Anxiety

This curriculum was developed as a training tool for pediatric continuity clinics to improve residency education regarding the assessment and management of anxiety in pediatrics (www.aap.org/en-us/advocacy-and-policy /aap-health-initiatives/Mental-Health/Pages/Module-2-Anxiety.aspx).

# Quality Ratings for Psychotherapies and Efficacy Data for Medications

## PracticeWise "Evidence-Based Child and Adolescent Psychosocial Interventions" Table

The PracticeWise "Evidence-Based Child and Adolescent Psychosocial Interventions" table summarizes evidence-based psychosocial interventions for youth. It is available at www.aap.org/en-us/Documents /CRPsychosocialInterventions.pdf and is updated every 6 months.

## Safety and Efficacy Studies Supporting Group 1 Medications (Table D-1)

As a proxy for the magnitude of effect, the rate of responders on active drug and placebo are listed. It is important to note that a responder is not the same as a remitter. A patient who remits no longer meets diagnostic criteria and has no or very mild residual symptoms, whereas a responder generally meets a severity criterion of "much better" or "very much better" but may still have mild to moderate symptoms. Thus, a remitter is generally more improved than a responder. The last column notes whether ratings were done by "independent evaluators" (IEs). An IE is a rater who is not involved in data collection other than to conduct blinded symptom severity ratings at specified times during a study. The use of IEs is thought to reduce bias because the presence or absence of medication adverse effects (which are reported to research clinicians but not to IEs) can help investigators guess the participant's medication status: active or placebo. Finally, all completed National Institute of Health–sponsored studies are included in the tables. However, there may be unpublished industry-sponsored studies that are not listed.

Table D-1. Evidence Supporting Short-term Safety and Efficacy of Group 1 Medications in Children and Adolescents

| Drug | Indication | Support | Age, years | Rate of Responders, % | IE[a] |
|---|---|---|---|---|---|
| Methylphenidate[b] | ADHD | Spencer et al (1996): Review[1] | 6–12 | A: approximately 70, P: approximately 25 | NA |
| | | MTA Cooperative Group (1999)[2] | 7–9 | Not specified | No |
| | | The PATS Team (2006)[3] | 3–5 | A: 21, P: 13 | No |
| Methylphenidate[c] | ADHD | Greenhill et al (2002)[4] | 6–16 | A: 64, P: 27 | No |
| | | McGough et al (2006): Patch[5] | 6–12 | A: 71, P: 16 | No |
| | | Findling et al (2010): Patch[6] | 13–17 | A: 66, P: 21 | No |
| Amphetamine[b] | ADHD | Spencer et al (1996): Review[1] | NA | NA | NA |
| Amphetamine[c] | ADHD | McGough et al (2005)[7] | 6–12 | Not specified | No |
| | | Domnitei and Madaan (2010)[8] | 6–12 | A: 70, P: 18 | No |
| Guanfacine[b] | ADHD | Scahill et al (2001)[9] | 7–15 | A: 53, P: 0 | No |
| | | Arnsten et al (2007): Review[10] | NA | NA | NA |
| Guanfacine[c] | ADHD | Biederman et al (2008)[11] | 6–17 | A: 50, P: 26 | No |
| | | Sallee et al (2009)[12] | 6–17 | A: 56, P: 30 | No |
| Clonidine[c] | ADHD | Jain et al (2011)[13] | 6–17 | NA | No |
| | | Kollins et al (2011)[14] | 6–17 | NA | No |
| Atomoxetine | ADHD | Michaelson et al (2001)[15] | 8–18 | Not specified | No |

| | | | | | |
|---|---|---|---|---|---|
| Fluoxetine | Anxiety | Birmaher et al (2003)[16] | 7–17 | A: 61, P: 35 | No |
| | MDD | Emslie et al (1997)[17] | 7–17 | A: 56, P: 33 | No |
| | | Emslie et al (2002)[18] | 8–18 | A: 65, P: 53 | No |
| | | March et al (2004)[19] | 12–17 | A: 61, P: 35 | Yes |
| | OCD | Riddle et al (1992)[20] | 8–15 | A: 33, P: 12 | No |
| | | Geller et al (2001)[21] | 7–17 | A: 49, P: 25 | No |
| | | Liebowitz et al (2002)[22] | 6–18 | A: 57, P: 27 | Yes |
| Sertraline | Anxiety | Walkup et al (2008)[23] | 7–17 | A: 55, P: 24 | Yes |
| | MDD | Wagner et al (2003)[24] | 6–17 | A: 36, P: 24 | No |
| | OCD | March et al (1998)[25] | 13–17 | A: 42, P: 26 | No |
| | | The POTS Team (2004)[26] | 7–17 | A: 21, P: 4 | Yes |
| Escitalopram | MDD | Wagner et al (2006)[27] | 6–17 | A: 63, P: 52 | No |
| | | Emslie et al (2009)[28] | 12–17 | A: 62, P: 52 | No |
| Fluvoxamine | Anxiety | RUPP Anxiety Group (2001)[29] | 6–17 | A: 76, P: 29 | No |
| | OCD | Riddle et al (2001)[30] | 8–17 | A: 42, P: 26 | No |

Abbreviations: A, active drug recipients; ADHD, attention-deficit/hyperactivity disorder; IE, independent evaluator; MDD, major depressive disorder; NA, not applicable; OCD, obsessive-compulsive disorder; P, placebo recipients.

[a] Use of IEs to rate symptom severity may help reduce bias because these individuals are blinded to patient adverse effects that could reveal their treatment assignment.

[b] Standard formulation.

[c] Extended-release formulation.

# References

1. Spencer T, Biederman J, Wilens T, Harding M, O'Donnell D, Griffin S. Pharmacotherapy of attention-deficit hyperactivity disorder across the life cycle. *J Am Acad Child Adolesc Psychiatry.* 1996;35(4):409–432

2. The MTA Cooperative Group. A 14-month randomized clinical trial of treatment strategies for attention-deficit/hyperactivity disorder: Multimodal Treatment Study of Children with ADHD. *Arch Gen Psychiatry.* 1999;56:1073–1086

3. Greenhill L, Kollins S, Abikoff H, et al. Efficacy and safety of immediate-release methylphenidate treatment for preschoolers with ADHD. *J Am Acad Child Adolesc Psychiatry.* 2006;45(11):1284–1293

4. Greenhill LL, Findling RL, Swanson JM; ADHD Study Group. A double-blind, placebo-controlled study of modified-release methylphenidate in children with attention-deficit/hyperactivity disorder. *Pediatrics.* 2002;109(3):E39

5. McGough JJ, Wigal SB, Abikoff H, Turnbow JM, Posner K, Moon E. A randomized, double-blind, placebo-controlled, laboratory classroom assessment of methylphenidate transdermal system in children with ADHD. *J Atten Disord.* 2006;9(3):476–485

6. Findling RL, Turnbow J, Burnside J, Melmed R, Civil R, Li Y. A randomized, double-blind, multicenter, parallel-group, placebo-controlled, dose-optimization study of the methylphenidate transdermal system for the treatment of ADHD in adolescents. *CNS Spectr.* 2010;15(7):419–430

7. McGough JJ, Biederman J, Wigal SB, et al. Long-term tolerability and effectiveness of once-daily mixed amphetamine salts (Adderall XR) in children with ADHD. *J Am Acad Child Adolesc Psychiatry.* 2005;44(6):530–538

8. Domnitei D, Madaan V. New and extended-action treatments in the management of ADHD: a critical appraisal of lisdexamfetamine in adults and children. *Neuropsychiatr Dis Treat.* 2010;6:273–279

9. Scahill L, Chappell PB, Kim YS, et al. A placebo-controlled study of guanfacine in the treatment of children with tic disorders and attention deficit hyperactivity disorder. *Am J Psychiatry.* 2001;158(7):1067–1074

10. Arnsten AF, Scahill L, Findling RL. alpha2-Adrenergic receptor agonists for the treatment of attention-deficit/hyperactivity disorder: emerging concepts from new data. *J Child Adolesc Psychopharmacol.* 2007;17(4):393–406

11. Biederman J, Melmed RD, Patel A, et al; SPD503 Study Group. A randomized, double-blind, placebo-controlled study of guanfacine extended release in children and adolescents with attention-deficit/hyperactivity disorder. *Pediatrics.* 2008;121(1):e73–e84

12. Sallee FR, McGough J, Wigal T, Donahue J, Lyne A, Biederman J; SPD503 Study Group. Guanfacine extended release in children and adolescents with attention-deficit/hyperactivity disorder: a placebo-controlled trial. *J Am Acad Child Adolesc Psychiatry.* 2009;48(2):155–165

13. Jain R, Segal S, Kollins SH, Khayrallah M. Clonidine extended-release tablets for pediatric patients with attention-deficit/hyperactivity disorder. *J Am Acad Child Adolesc Psychiatry.* 2011;50(2):171–179

14. Kollins SH, Jain R, Brams M, et al. Clonidine extended-release tablets as add-on therapy to psychostimulants in children and adolescents with ADHD. *Pediatrics.* 2011;127(6):e1406–e1413

15. Michelson D, Faries D, Wernicke J, et al; Atomoxetine ADHD Study Group. Atomoxetine in the treatment of children and adolescents with attention-deficit/hyperactivity disorder: a randomized, placebo-controlled, dose-response study. *Pediatrics.* 2001; 108(5):E83

16. Birmaher B, Axelson DA, Monk K, et al. Fluoxetine for the treatment of childhood anxiety disorders. *J Am Acad Child Adolesc Psychiatry.* 2003;42:415–423

17. Emslie GJ, Rush AJ, Weinberg WA, et al. A double-blind, randomized, placebo-controlled trial of fluoxetine in children and adolescents with depression. *Arch Gen Psychiatry.* 1997;54(11):1031–1037

18. Emslie GJ, Heiligenstein JH, Wagner KD, et al. Fluoxetine for acute treatment of depression in children and adolescents: a placebo-controlled, randomized clinical trial. *J Am Acad Child Adolesc Psychiatry.* 2002;41(10):1205–1215

19. March J, Silva S, Petrycki S, et al. Fluoxetine, cognitive-behavioral therapy, and their combination for adolescents with depression: treatment for Adolescents With Depression Study (TADS) randomized controlled trial. *JAMA.* 2004;292:807–820

20. Riddle MA, Scahill L, King RA, et al. Double-blind, crossover trial of fluoxetine and placebo in children and adolescents with obsessive-compulsive disorder. *J Am Acad Child Adolesc Psychiatry.* 1992;31(6):1062–1069

21. Geller DA, Hoog SL, Heiligenstein JH, et al; Fluoxetine Pediatric OCD Study Team. Fluoxetine treatment for obsessive-compulsive disorder in children and adolescents: a placebo-controlled clinical trial. *J Am Acad Child Adolesc Psychiatry.* 2001;40(7):773–779

22. Liebowitz MR, Turner SM, Piacentini J, et al. Fluoxetine in children and adolescents with OCD: a placebo-controlled trial. *J Am Acad Child Adolesc Psychiatry.* 2002;41(12): 1431–1438

23. Walkup JT, Albano AM, Piacentini J, et al. Cognitive behavioral therapy, sertraline, or a combination in childhood anxiety. *N Engl J Med.* 2008;359:2753–2766

24. Wagner KD, Ambrosini P, Rynn M, et al; Sertraline Pediatric Depression Study Group. Efficacy of sertraline in the treatment of children and adolescents with major depressive disorder: two randomized controlled trials. *JAMA.* 2003;290(8):1033–1041

25. March JS, Biederman J, Wolkow R, et al. Sertraline in children and adolescents with obsessive-compulsive disorder: a multicenter randomized controlled trial. *JAMA.* 1998;280(20):1752–1756

26. Pediatric OCD Treatment Study (POTS) Team. Cognitive-behavior therapy, sertraline, and their combination for children and adolescents with obsessive-compulsive disorder: the Pediatric OCD Treatment Study (POTS) randomized controlled trial. *JAMA.* 2004;292(16):1969–1976

27. Wagner KD, Jonas J, Findling RL, Ventura D, Saikali K. A double-blind, randomized, placebo-controlled trial of escitalopram in the treatment of pediatric depression. *J Am Acad Child Adolesc Psychiatry.* 2006;45(3):280–288

28. Emslie GJ, Ventura D, Korotzer A, Tourkodimitris S. Escitalopram in the treatment of adolescent depression: a randomized placebo-controlled multisite trial. *J Am Acad Child Adolesc Psychiatry.* 2009;48(7):721–729

29. The Research Unit on Pediatric Psychopharmacology Anxiety Study Group. Fluvoxamine for the treatment of anxiety disorders in children and adolescents. *N Engl J Med.* 2001;344:1279–1785

30. Riddle MA, Reeve EA, Yaryura-Tobias JA, et al. Fluvoxamine for children and adolescents with obsessive-compulsive disorder: a randomized, controlled, multicenter trial. *J Am Acad Child Adolesc Psychiatry.* 2001;40(2):222–229

# Resources for Caregivers

## American Academy of Pediatrics Resources

### Books
- *Mental Health, Naturally: The Family Guide to Holistic Care for a Healthy Mind and Body* by Kathi J. Kemper, MD, FAAP
- *ADHD: What Every Parent Needs to Know*, 2nd Edition, edited by Michael I. Reiff, MD, FAAP
- *Autism Spectrum Disorders: What Every Parent Needs to Know* edited by Alan I. Rosenblatt, MD, FAAP, and Paul S. Carbone, MD, FAAP

### Patient Education Brochures (http://patiented.solutions.aap.org)
- *Understanding Autism Spectrum Disorders (ASDs)*
- *Your Child's Mental Health*
- *Teen Suicide*

### Web Sites
- **HealthyChildren.org:** HealthyChildren.org is the only parenting Web site backed by 64,000 pediatricians committed to the attainment of optimal physical, mental, and social health and well-being for all infants, children, adolescents, and young adults.

## Facts for Families

The American Academy of Child and Adolescent Psychiatry's *Facts for Families* provide concise and up-to-date information on issues that affect children, teenagers, and their families. AACAP provides this important information as a public service. The *Facts for Families* may be duplicated and distributed free of charge as long as the American Academy of Child and

Adolescent Psychiatry is properly credited and no profit is gained from their use. (https://www.aacap.org/aacap/Families_and_Youth/Facts_for_Families /Facts_for_Families_Keyword.aspx)

# National Federation of Families for Children's Mental Health

The National Federation of Families for Children's Mental Health is a national family-run organization linking more than 120 chapters and state organizations focused on the issues of children and youth with emotional, behavioral, or mental health needs and their families. The National Federation works to develop and implement policies, legislation, funding mechanisms, and service systems that utilize the strengths of families. Its emphasis on advocacy offers families a voice in the formation of national policy, services, and supports for children with mental health needs and their families.

# Johns Hopkins University Center for Mental Health Services in Pediatric Primary Care

The Johns Hopkins University Center for Mental Health Services in Pediatric Primary Care (http://web.jhu.edu/pedmentalhealth) is a resource for primary care clinicians. The center focuses on discovery and dissemination of evidence-based assessments and treatments. The author of this book (Dr Riddle) and 2 contributing editors (Drs Pruitt and Wissow) are faculty members of the center.

# US FDA Package Inserts

A "Patient Counseling Information" or "Medication Guide" section can be found at the end of US Food and Drug Administration package inserts. They should be given to the patient at the pharmacy or via mail. To see an example of a US Food and Drug Administration package insert, visit www.accessdata .fda.gov/drugsatfda_docs/label/2011/018936s091lbl.pdf.

# Diagnostic and Statistical Manual of Mental Disorders, Fifth Edition, Complete Criteria of Select Diagnoses

## Attention-Deficit/Hyperactivity Disorder

### Diagnostic Criteria

A. A persistent pattern of inattention and/or hyperactivity-impulsivity that interferes with functioning or development, as characterized by (1) and/or (2):

1. **Inattention:** Six (or more) of the following symptoms have persisted for at least 6 months to a degree that is inconsistent with developmental level and that negatively impacts directly on social and academic/occupational activities:
   **Note:** The symptoms are not solely a manifestation of oppositional behavior, defiance, hostility, or failure to understand tasks or instructions. For older adolescents and adults (age 17 and older), at least five symptoms are required.

   a. Often fails to give close attention to details or makes careless mistakes in schoolwork, at work, or during other activities (e.g., overlooks or misses details, work is inaccurate).

   b. Often has difficulty sustaining attention in tasks or play activities (e.g., has difficulty remaining focused during lectures, conversations, or lengthy reading).

   c. Often does not seem to listen when spoken to directly (e.g., mind seems elsewhere, even in the absence of any obvious distraction).

   d. Often does not follow through on instructions and fails to finish schoolwork, chores, or duties in the workplace (e.g., starts tasks but quickly loses focus and is easily sidetracked).

   e. Often has difficulty organizing tasks and activities (e.g., difficulty managing sequential tasks; difficulty keeping materials and belongings in order; messy, disorganized work; has poor time management; fails to meet deadlines).

   f. Often avoids, dislikes, or is reluctant to engage in tasks that require sustained mental effort (e.g., schoolwork or homework; for older adolescents and adults, preparing reports, completing forms, reviewing lengthy papers).

   g. Often loses things necessary for tasks or activities (e.g., school materials, pencils, books, tools, wallets, keys, paperwork, eyeglasses, mobile telephones).

   h. Is often easily distracted by extraneous stimuli (for older adolescents and adults, may include unrelated thoughts).

   i. Is often forgetful in daily activities (e.g., doing chores, running errands; for older adolescents and adults, returning calls, paying bills, keeping appointments).

2. **Hyperactivity and impulsivity:** Six (or more) of the following symptoms have persisted for at least 6 months to a degree that is inconsistent with developmental level and that negatively impacts directly on social and academic/occupational activities: **Note:** The symptoms are not solely a manifestation of oppositional behavior, defiance, hostility, or a failure to understand tasks or instructions. For older adolescents and adults (age 17 and older), at least five symptoms are required.

   a. Often fidgets with or taps hands or feet or squirms in seat.
   b. Often leaves seat in situations when remaining seated is expected (e.g., leaves his or her place in the classroom, in the office or other workplace, or in other situations that require remaining in place).
   c. Often runs about or climbs in situations where it is inappropriate. (**Note:** In adolescents or adults, may be limited to feeling restless.)
   d. Often unable to play or engage in leisure activities quietly.
   e. Is often "on the go," acting as if "driven by a motor" (e.g., is unable to be or uncomfortable being still for extended time, as in restaurants, meetings; may be experienced by others as being restless or difficult to keep up with).
   f. Often talks excessively.
   g. Often blurts out an answer before a question has been completed (e.g., completes people's sentences; cannot wait for turn in conversation).
   h. Often has difficulty waiting his or her turn (e.g., while waiting in line).
   i. Often interrupts or intrudes on others (e.g., butts into conversations, games, or activities; may start using other people's things without asking or receiving permission; for adolescents and adults, may intrude into or take over what others are doing).

B. Several inattentive or hyperactive-impulsive symptoms were present prior to age 12 years.

C. Several inattentive or hyperactive-impulsive symptoms are present in two or more settings (e.g., at home, school, or work; with friends or relatives; in other activities).

D. There is clear evidence that the symptoms interfere with, or reduce the quality of, social, academic, or occupational functioning.

E. The symptoms do not occur exclusively during the course of schizophrenia or another psychotic disorder and are not better explained by another mental disorder (e.g., mood disorder, anxiety disorder, dissociative disorder, personality disorder, substance intoxication or withdrawal).

*Specify* whether:

**314.01 (F90.2) Combined presentation:** If both Criterion A1 (inattention) and Criterion A2 (hyperactivity-impulsivity) are met for the past 6 months.

**314.00 (F90.0) Predominantly inattentive presentation:** If Criterion A1 (inattention) is met but Criterion A2 (hyperactivity-impulsivity) is not met for the past 6 months.

**314.01 (F90.1) Predominantly hyperactive/impulsive presentation:** If Criterion A2 (hyperactivity-impulsivity) is met and Criterion A1 (inattention) is not met for the past 6 months.

*Specify* if:

**in partial remission:** When full criteria were previously met, fewer than the full criteria have been met for the past 6 months, and the symptoms still result in impairment in social, academic, or occupational functioning.

*Specify* current severity:

**Mild:** Few, if any, symptoms in excess of those required to make the diagnosis are present, and symptoms result in no more than minor impairments in social or occupational functioning.

**Moderate:** Symptoms or functional impairment between "mild" and "severe" are present.

**Severe:** Many symptoms in excess of those required to make the diagnosis, or several symptoms that are particularly severe, are present, or the symptoms result in marked impairment in social or occupational functioning.

# Disruptive Mood Dysregulation Disorder

Diagnostic Criteria                                    **296.99 (F34.8)**

A. Severe recurrent temper outbursts manifested verbally (e.g., verbal rages) and/or behaviorally (e.g., physical aggression toward people or property) that are grossly out of proportion in intensity or duration to the situation or provocation.
B. The temper outbursts are inconsistent with developmental level.
C. The temper outbursts occur, on average, three or more times per week.
D. The mood between temper outbursts is persistently irritable or angry most of the day, nearly every day, and is observable by others (e.g., parents, teachers, peers).
E. Criteria A–D have been present for 12 or more months. Throughout that time, the individual has not had a period lasting 3 or more consecutive months without all of the symptoms in Criteria A–D.
F. Criteria A and D are present in at least two of three settings (i.e., at home, at school, with peers) and are severe in at least one of these.
G. The diagnosis should not be made for the first time before age 6 years or after age 18 years.
H. By history or observation, the age at onset of Criteria A–E is before 10 years.
I. There has never been a distinct period lasting more than 1 day during which the full symptom criteria, except duration, for a manic or hypomanic episode have been met.
   **Note:** Developmentally appropriate mood elevation, such as occurs in the context of a highly positive event or its anticipation, should not be considered as a symptom of mania or hypomania.
J. The behaviors do not occur exclusively during an episode of major depressive disorder and are not better explained by another mental disorder (e.g., autism spectrum disorder, posttraumatic stress disorder, separation anxiety disorder, persistent depressive disorder [dysthymia]).
   **Note:** This diagnosis cannot coexist with oppositional defiant disorder, intermittent explosive disorder, or bipolar disorder, though it can coexist with others, including major depressive disorder, attention-deficit/hyperactivity disorder, conduct disorder, and substance use disorders. Individuals whose symptoms meet criteria for both disruptive mood dysregulation disorder and oppositional defiant disorder should only be given the diagnosis of disruptive mood dysregulation disorder. If an individual has ever experienced a manic or hypomanic episode, the diagnosis of disruptive mood dysregulation disorder should not be assigned.
K. The symptoms are not attributable to the physiological effects of a substance or to another medical or neurological condition.

# Generalized Anxiety Disorder

## Diagnostic Criteria                                    300.02 (F41.1)

A. Excessive anxiety and worry (apprehensive expectation), occurring more days than not for at least 6 months, about a number of events or activities (such as work or school performance).

B. The individual finds it difficult to control the worry.

C. The anxiety and worry are associated with three (or more) of the following six symptoms (with at least some symptoms having been present for more days than not for the past 6 months):

**Note:** Only one item is required in children.

1. Restlessness or feeling keyed up or on edge.
2. Being easily fatigued.
3. Difficulty concentrating or mind going blank.
4. Irritability.
5. Muscle tension.
6. Sleep disturbance (difficulty falling or staying asleep, or restless, unsatisfying sleep).

D. The anxiety, worry, or physical symptoms cause clinically significant distress or impairment in social, occupational, or other important areas of functioning.

E. The disturbance is not attributable to the physiological effects of a substance (e.g., a drug of abuse, a medication) or another medical condition (e.g., hyperthyroidism).

F. The disturbance is not better explained by another mental disorder (e.g., anxiety or worry about having panic attacks in panic disorder, negative evaluation in social anxiety disorder [social phobia], contamination or other obsessions in obsessive-compulsive disorder, separation from attachment figures in separation anxiety disorder, reminders of traumatic events in posttraumatic stress disorder, gaining weight in anorexia nervosa, physical complaints in somatic symptom disorder, perceived appearance flaws in body dysmorphic disorder, having a serious illness in illness anxiety disorder, or the content of delusional beliefs in schizophrenia or delusional disorder).

# Major Depressive Disorder

## Diagnostic Criteria

A. Five (or more) of the following symptoms have been present during the same 2-week period and represent a change from previous functioning; at least one of the symptoms is either (1) depressed mood or (2) loss of interest or pleasure.

**Note:** Do not include symptoms that are clearly attributable to another medical condition.

1. Depressed mood most of the day, nearly every day, as indicated by either subjective report (e.g., feels sad, empty, hopeless) or observation made by others (e.g., appears tearful). (**Note:** In children and adolescents, can be irritable mood.)
2. Markedly diminished interest or pleasure in all, or almost all, activities most of the day, nearly every day (as indicated by either subjective account or observation).

3. Significant weight loss when not dieting or weight gain (e.g., a change of more than 5% of body weight in a month), or decrease or increase in appetite nearly every day. (**Note:** In children, consider failure to make expected weight gain.)

4. Insomnia or hypersomnia nearly every day.

5. Psychomotor agitation or retardation nearly every day (observable by others, not merely subjective feelings of restlessness or being slowed down).

6. Fatigue or loss of energy nearly every day.

7. Feelings of worthlessness or excessive or inappropriate guilt (which may be delusional) nearly every day (not merely self-reproach or guilt about being sick).

8. Diminished ability to think or concentrate, or indecisiveness, nearly every day (either by subjective account or as observed by others).

9. Recurrent thoughts of death (not just fear of dying), recurrent suicidal ideation without a specific plan, or a suicide attempt or a specific plan for committing suicide.

B. The symptoms cause clinically significant distress or impairment in social, occupational, or other important areas of functioning.

C. The episode is not attributable to the physiological effects of a substance or to another medical condition.

**Note:** Criteria A–C represent a major depressive episode.

**Note:** Responses to a significant loss (e.g., bereavement, financial ruin, losses from a natural disaster, a serious medical illness or disability) may include the feelings of intense sadness, rumination about the loss, insomnia, poor appetite, and weight loss noted in Criterion A, which may resemble a depressive episode. Although such symptoms may be understandable or considered appropriate to the loss, the presence of a major depressive episode in addition to the normal response to a significant loss should also be carefully considered. This decision inevitably requires the exercise of clinical judgment based on the individual's history and the cultural norms for the expression of distress in the context of loss.[1]

D. The occurrence of the major depressive episode is not better explained by schizoaffective disorder, schizophrenia, schizophreniform disorder, delusional disorder, or other specified and unspecified schizophrenia spectrum and other psychotic disorders.

E. There has never been a manic episode or a hypomanic episode.

**Note:** This exclusion does not apply if all of the manic-like or hypomanic-like episodes are substance-induced or are attributable to the physiological effects of another medical condition.

---

[1] In distinguishing grief from a major depressive episode (MDE), it is useful to consider that in grief the predominant affect is feelings of emptiness and loss, while in MDE it is persistent depressed mood and the inability to anticipate happiness or pleasure. The dysphoria in grief is likely to decrease in intensity over days to weeks and occurs in waves, the so-called pangs of grief. These waves tend to be associated with thoughts or reminders of the deceased. The depressed mood of MDE is more persistent and not tied to specific thoughts or preoccupations. The pain of grief may be accompanied by positive emotions and humor that are uncharacteristic of the pervasive unhappiness and misery characteristic of MDE. The thought content associated with grief generally features a preoccupation with thoughts and memories of the deceased, rather than the self-critical or pessimistic ruminations seen in MDE. In grief, self-esteem is generally preserved, whereas in MDE feelings of worthlessness and self-loathing are common. If self-derogatory ideation is present in grief, it typically involves perceived failings vis-à-vis the deceased (e.g., not visiting frequently enough, not telling the deceased how much he or she was loved). If a bereaved individual thinks about death and dying, such thoughts are generally focused on the deceased and possibly about "joining" the deceased, whereas in MDE such thoughts are focused on ending one's own life because of feeling worthless, undeserving of life, or unable to cope with the pain of depression.

### Coding and Recording Procedures

The diagnostic code for major depressive disorder is based on whether this is a single or recurrent episode, current severity, presence of psychotic features, and remission status. Current severity and psychotic features are only indicated if full criteria are currently met for a major depressive episode. Remission specifiers are only indicated if the full criteria are not currently met for a major depressive episode. Codes are as follows:

| Severity/course specifier | Single episode | Recurrent episode* |
|---|---|---|
| Mild (p. 188) | 296.21 (F32.0) | 296.31 (F33.0) |
| Moderate (p. 188) | 296.22 (F32.1) | 296.32 (F33.1) |
| Severe (p. 188) | 296.23 (F32.2) | 296.33 (F33.2) |
| With psychotic features** (p. 186) | 296.24 (F32.3) | 296.34 (F33.3) |
| In partial remission (p. 188) | 296.25 (F32.4) | 296.35 (F33.41) |
| In full remission (p. 188) | 296.26 (F32.5) | 296.36 (F33.42) |
| Unspecified | 296.20 (F32.9) | 296.30 (F33.9) |

*For an episode to be considered recurrent, there must be an interval of at least 2 consecutive months between separate episodes in which criteria are not met for a major depressive episode. The definitions of specifiers are found on the indicated pages.
**If psychotic features are present, code the "with psychotic features" specifier irrespective of episode severity.

Reprinted with permission from the Diagnostic and Statistical Manual of Mental Disorders, Fifth Edition, (Copyright 2013). American Psychiatric Association.

# Oppositional Defiant Disorder

## Diagnostic Criteria                                         313.81 (F91.3)

A.  A pattern of angry/irritable mood, argumentative/defiant behavior, or vindictiveness lasting at least 6 months as evidenced by at least four symptoms from any of the following categories, and exhibited during interaction with at least one individual who is not a sibling.

### Angry/Irritable Mood

1.  Often loses temper.
2.  Is often touchy or easily annoyed.
3.  Is often angry and resentful.

### Argumentative/Defiant Behavior

4.  Often argues with authority figures or, for children and adolescents, with adults.
5.  Often actively defies or refuses to comply with requests from authority figures or with rules.
6.  Often deliberately annoys others.
7.  Often blames others for his or her mistakes or misbehavior.

### Vindictiveness

8.  Has been spiteful or vindictive at least twice within the past 6 months.

**Note:** The persistence and frequency of these behaviors should be used to distinguish a behavior that is within normal limits from a behavior that is symptomatic. For children younger than 5 years, the behavior should occur on most days for a period of at least 6 months unless otherwise noted (Criterion A8). For individuals 5 years or older, the behavior should occur at least once per week for at least 6 months, unless otherwise noted (Criterion A8). While these frequency criteria provide guidance on a minimal level of frequency to define symptoms, other factors should also be considered, such as whether the frequency and intensity of the behaviors are outside a range that is normative for the individual's developmental level, gender, and culture.

B. The disturbance in behavior is associated with distress in the individual or others in his or her immediate social context (e.g., family, peer group, work colleagues), or it impacts negatively on social, educational, occupational, or other important areas of functioning.

C. The behaviors do not occur exclusively during the course of a psychotic, substance use, depressive, or bipolar disorder. Also, the criteria are not met for disruptive mood dysregulation disorder.

*Specify* current severity:

**Mild:** Symptoms are confined to only one setting (e.g., at home, at school, at work, with peers).

**Moderate:** Some symptoms are present in at least two settings.

**Severe:** Some symptoms are present in three or more settings.

# Separation Anxiety Disorder

## Diagnostic Criteria      309.21 (F93.0)

A. Developmentally inappropriate and excessive fear or anxiety concerning separation from those to whom the individual is attached, as evidenced by at least three of the following:

1. Recurrent excessive distress when anticipating or experiencing separation from home or from major attachment figures.

2. Persistent and excessive worry about losing major attachment figures or about possible harm to them, such as illness, injury, disasters, or death.

3. Persistent and excessive worry about experiencing an untoward event (e.g., getting lost, being kidnapped, having an accident, becoming ill) that causes separation from a major attachment figure.

4. Persistent reluctance or refusal to go out, away from home, to school, to work, or elsewhere because of fear of separation.

5. Persistent and excessive fear of or reluctance about being alone or without major attachment figures at home or in other settings.

6. Persistent reluctance or refusal to sleep away from home or to go to sleep without being near a major attachment figure.

7. Repeated nightmares involving the theme of separation.

8. Repeated complaints of physical symptoms (e.g., headaches, stomachaches, nausea, vomiting) when separation from major attachment figures occurs or is anticipated.

B. The fear, anxiety, or avoidance is persistent, lasting at least 4 weeks in children and adolescents and typically 6 months or more in adults.

C. The disturbance causes clinically significant distress or impairment in social, academic, occupational, or other important areas of functioning.

D. The disturbance is not better explained by another mental disorder, such as refusing to leave home because of excessive resistance to change in autism spectrum disorder; delusions or hallucinations concerning separation in psychotic disorders; refusal to go outside without a trusted companion in agoraphobia; worries about ill health or other harm befalling significant others in generalized anxiety disorder; or concerns about having an illness in illness anxiety disorder.

# Social Anxiety Disorder (Social Phobia)

## Diagnostic Criteria                    300.23 (F40.10)

A. Marked fear or anxiety about one or more social situations in which the individual is exposed to possible scrutiny by others. Examples include social interactions (e.g., having a conversation, meeting unfamiliar people), being observed (e.g., eating or drinking), and performing in front of others (e.g., giving a speech).

**Note:** In children, the anxiety must occur in peer settings and not just during interactions with adults.

B. The individual fears that he or she will act in a way or show anxiety symptoms that will be negatively evaluated (i.e., will be humiliating or embarrassing; will lead to rejection or offend others).

C. The social situations almost always provoke fear or anxiety.

**Note:** In children, the fear or anxiety may be expressed by crying, tantrums, freezing, clinging, shrinking, or failing to speak in social situations.

D. The social situations are avoided or endured with intense fear or anxiety.

E. The fear or anxiety is out of proportion to the actual threat posed by the social situation and to the sociocultural context.

F. The fear, anxiety, or avoidance is persistent, typically lasting for 6 months or more.

G. The fear, anxiety, or avoidance causes clinically significant distress or impairment in social, occupational, or other important areas of functioning.

H. The fear, anxiety, or avoidance is not attributable to the physiological effects of a substance (e.g., a drug of abuse, a medication) or another medical condition.

I. The fear, anxiety, or avoidance is not better explained by the symptoms of another mental disorder, such as panic disorder, body dysmorphic disorder, or autism spectrum disorder.

J. If another medical condition (e.g., Parkinson's disease, obesity, disfigurement from burns or injury) is present, the fear, anxiety, or avoidance is clearly unrelated or is excessive.

*Specify* if:

**Performance only:** If the fear is restricted to speaking or performing in public.

# Index

Page numbers in *italic* denote a figure, table, or box.